MW01035513

The Ultimate Guide to Life for
Fatherless Teenage Boys:

What Our Father Wants Me To Tell You

Michael W. Newman

A Man's Legacy Press
KDP Print & E-Book Edition
©2019

Please contact the author at:
MNewman4321@yahoo.com

DEDICATION

I am dedicating this book to my two brothers, David ("Tuber") and Sean ("Filbert") Newman, both younger than me. Not because they were always great, awesome, and fun brothers to be with when we were growing up. They weren't. Not in the slightest. We didn't always get along, that's for sure. We fought, we argued, we despised one another (at times). Rather, I am dedicating this book to them because, like me (the author), they, too, grew up fatherless. And despite the long odds being against them, they overcame the tough obstacles and became honest, true, and loyal fathers themselves to their own beautiful, incredible sons. That, to me, is just amazing. A heaven-sent miracle. Beyond any words I can write in this short paragraph adequately. That is why I choose to honor my wonderful brothers here, now and always. *You rock, David and Sean!!!*

*You rock, too, my dear sister, Tricia, for being the fantastic mother you are. But this book is for boys only. Hopefully some fatherless woman will get the inspiration and step up to write a book like this one for fatherless girls

A QUICK MESSAGE

To David's son, Cool Max...

To Sean's son, Funny Simon...

To my son, Awesome Mikey...

Sorry we have failed you so many times as your fathers and uncles. Just know that we are trying the best we can, with what we have, to give you better childhoods and teenage years than we had ourselves.

"Society asks if there is any hope for me. I say 'yes'. Why? Because I live content in God's Grace. After all, who put my dumb ass in prison? If I wanted a better life for myself, I should have made better decisions."

JEREMY BRUCE SLY
Fatherless at age 5
Homeless runaway at age 14
Sentenced to life without parole in
Florida Prison at age 22
Committed his life to Christ at age 39
"Reborn"

TABLE OF CONTENTS

FOREWARD

May the Lord find me a positive male pro-athlete to write a preface to be placed here as inspiration to the young boys this book is intended for.

INTRODUCTION

Why did you write this book, Mr. Michael?

I wrote this book for you, my little friend, because I care for you. I may never meet you, but I wish I could! I wrote it because I was once right there, right where you are today. You might call me a 'born-loser' who didn't figure out the good ideas written in this book until I was in my 30s and already married - very late in life I must reluctantly admit. Yes, I was hard-headed and ignorant for far too long. And now I want to help you and protect you, little brother, while it can still be easy for you to change your circumstances. I want you to know that you are not forever 'stuck' where you are right now. I want you to know that life is full of decisions, and that positive changes can happen if you put your own efforts and faith into them.

That's why I wrote this book. *For you to become a better person, for you to grow up to become a man of God.* Life is short. Keep it simple and beautiful and the world will be at your feet. There are unlimited possibilities in your life. You are a child of God, and you have every right to be here and make your life what you will as best as you can.

One thing to note: As you are reading, you will probably say, "Mr. Michael, you already mentioned that idea a few pages (or a chapter) ago! Why are you repeating it here again?"

Well, little friend, I am not very good with analogies, as my 10th grade biology teacher will surely tell you, but let me try to explain here why I repeat ideas so many times in this book:

I don't want you to think of the ideas and concepts in this book to be like 'hamburgers' that you eat one and move on to the next one in line, one at a time. Rather the ideas and concepts, as you read them, are more like a 'stack of pancakes', where, when you take a bite, you are biting a part of the entire 'stack of ideas'. Many ideas are presented all at the same time in one chapter, and then repeated in different places in other chapters, because the ideas overlap in the many important areas discussed in this book. Understanding the overlap of ideas is key to understanding this book. Also, some of this book doesn't apply to your age right now. Some of the information here is helpful for you today; other parts will help you later in future years.

You will read words like "change", "decisions", "potential", "consequences/results", "future", "good", "meaning", "faith", and "Godly" many times in this book. I hope you will be able to understand why I use these words frequently and what each of them means.

Lastly, when I sat down to start writing this book, I promised myself that it would not be 'preachy' to you in any way. I am not a minister, preacher, priest, or any other type of clergy that can answer any or all of your questions about God and religion adequately. And I won't pretend to, either. This book is indeed based on Christian principles that I have come to know to be true and right, yes. But also I am grateful to my good male friends who are not Christian (such as my Muslim or Agnostic friends) who gave me important and needed coaching, advice, and ideas to place in this book. To go further with this notion: there were even many contemporary Christian men I reached out to for help with this book who ignored and didn't even care to acknowledge my multiple requests for assistance or advice, for reasons I don't really quite understand. Many of them are fathers themselves, too. Go figure.

Chapter I - It's Not Your Fault

Let's try something here that you definitely need to do, because I one time needed to do it, too:

Get angry, little man. I mean *get really angry*. Feel it! Why? The fact is unmistakable: you are *pissed* and *hurt* that you don't have a father. And there is no way for us to move forward together until you deal with your negative emotions. You have every right to be angry for not having a father. But as you get angry, say this following sentence in front of a mirror.

"It's not your fault you don't have a father!"

Go ahead and read that again, little brother. That's my opening encouragement to you as we begin a journey in this book of understanding ourselves – you and me, boys without fathers – and the lives we will live better if we give ourselves the chance to make positive changes.

Repeat the paraphrased title of this chapter this way, loudly and boldly as often as you need to:

"It's NOT my fault I don't have a father!"
Say that in front of a mirror every morning and evening for ten days in a row, and I guarantee you will see a significant change in how you view yourself and your situation in life.

If you get only one idea from this book, let it be that phrase. (But I hope you get more from this book than just that phrase.) Repeat it every morning when you get up from bed and repeat it every evening before you go to sleep for the night.

"But why should I believe that?"

Believe it because it's true - not just because some guy you will probably never know, or meet is writing a book telling you to believe it - and it will change you for good forever. It's not your fault in any way, shape, or form that you don't have a father. Nobody, not a single person, in this world believes that it is your fault, either. You need to believe that sentence in your head and your heart yourself before any other positive changes in your life can be made. Until you accept that your fatherlessness is NOT your fault, you are going to be in serious spiritual pain and struggle emotionally all of your days and nights for now and always. And no good change ever happens in this worldly life for a young man who continues to endure such long-lasting pain because he has the misfortune of believing that it is his fault he is fatherless. It just doesn't happen. Believe it, because it is true. Trust me, little brother, because I've lived it, and I lived it for far too long. Overcome this idea, I beg you to. It's indeed what is best for you.

"Okay, I said it. But why then am I fatherless?"

I don't why you not having a father happened to you. Maybe your father died young. Maybe he left your mother (and you and your other brothers and sisters) stranded and abandoned and didn't care enough to come back. Maybe your mother doesn't even know who your father is. God, however, does not make 'accidents'. There is probably no one alive who can give you the right answer or a 'good enough' response that will satisfy your desire to answer the question why you don't have a father. There are a lot of questions on earth we won't know or understand the answers to until we die and go to heaven. I won't lie to you: it will be hard here for a while in your life at least. But your personal stability depends on you having to accept that you don't have a father and that it isn't in any way your fault. Dwelling on '*Why?*' will get you nowhere fast. Accept it and move forward.

"So how can I move on from this bad situation I am in?"

Moving onward for the chance at a better life at this point gives you two choices: you can wallow in self-pity and play the victim, thus you yourself choosing to make your own life miserable and devoid ever of anything fun or productive, OR you can choose to devote yourself to making the best of your situation (with all that you do have positively going for you) and vowing not to let this same catastrophic situation happen to your own son (should you have one) someday. Somehow, someway, you can, and you will, if you want to, make something positive out of this bad situation. You can, and you will, if you put your heart, mind, and soul into it. God says in the bible He can make good come out of anything bad. How about a flow-chart of this? Quickly write down on a blank piece of paper what goodness you'd like to see for your own son someday and then write down what it takes to get that positive life for your son, and then write down just next to that how you can possibly obtain the same things for yourself right now without the help of a father. Do you see a pattern here? Unfortunately, much of what you want and need in life right now as a young teenager could best come from having a father to support you and love you, but as we will see in a later chapter, another man can be an adequate (though not perfect!) substitution for your missing father.

I have nothing to gain by lying to you, little brother. My concern is not only for you as an individual, but also all boys like you in the same situation of fatherlessness. And there are many, many boys like you. Millions of North American boys grow up fatherless. Even beyond such horrible issues as racism and poverty, fatherlessness is the worst social crisis we have in the United States. Black American boys, White American boys, Asian American boys, Latino American boys. Privileged rich boys or desperately poor boys. These criteria don't change the effects of fatherlessness. It's even a problem throughout the whole world, getting worse and worse as history moves on. So, you are by far not all alone in this awful mess you are in.

I, the author of this book, was fatherless, too, growing up, as were my two younger brothers and one younger sister. Ignore me and what is written in this book here because what I say is unwelcome, tough to accept, and because it will take effort and be difficult to apply to your own life, and you'll be ignoring a grown man who was once your age and made a lot of bad, stupid mistakes because my growing up fatherless led me to. To ignore the advice, experience, and knowledge that can help you completely remake your life's direction better now and, in the future, can be, in a word, just *stupid.*

Not having a father is a terrible thing, but most people are missing something in their life. An awful thing to miss is a mother's love, especially when the mother is present. That kind of 'missing' few others around a boy can see. But if it is your case, then you know it, and sometimes only you know it, and it hurts bad. In another scenario, what if you had a father but were missing a leg, or an eye, or a sound mind? Would that be a better life? Strange as it may sound, a missing father has one advantage: you'll never have to depend on him or be surprised when he doesn't deliver. He will never let you down again, because he can't let you down again. Something also worse than not having a father is having one that everyone thinks is great and perfect, but the son knows that the truth and reality of it are different and aren't pretty (such as the verbal or physical abuse he could be suffering from his father).

Whatever happened to make you fatherless happened in the past. It is done, it is finished, and now it is up to you to press onward and upward, into the future. As said above, it's is impossible for your father to let you down again. Admitted honestly, the past let-down was huge and painful, but at least it's over, if you will let it be over. Learn to deal with it. Accept it with boldness of heart. If you hold blame against your missing father in your heart and you are right, what does that achieve? Look forward. You don't know what is in the future. You can only know what is in the past, however hazy that hindsight is.

Make forgiveness of your father a centerpiece of your being. This is crucial to your well-being. If you don't forgive your father for not being there for you, no matter the reason why he isn't there for you, you will remain bitter and emotionally sick about it all your life. You also will develop an unhealthy mistrust of all other men. This can only hold you back from potential future improvement in your situation because rightly, so you will definitely need other men in your life.

Ultimately, as you will see at the end of this book, being truly 'fatherless' is a choice every young boy (and older man) makes, because we all as human beings have the option to accept God as our One, True Father. If we fail to accept God into our lives, in that case, we are thus 'fatherless' on earth only by our own misdirected choice.

Chapter II - The First Step

You've gotten this far in the book, great, little brother! It shows that you care enough about yourself that you want changes in your life. So, what happens now that I have your full attention? Let's get angry again. Yes, get angry! Loudly! Feel it!

"God, I am angry at you because you didn't give me the father I want!"

Admit this anger, too, because it is real, so you can move on. It's okay to be angry at God, little brother. Really. He can take it, and He will make you better for it when you admit it honestly to Him. That's a fact you can believe in.

Right now, at this very moment, I bet you would trade anything you own to have someone just give you a few minutes of their time and listen to you. Especially, you would love for an older man to listen to you. That, my little friend, is something I would bet my whole savings account on, because I am so sure of it!

It is said that a real father does three things for his sons (and daughters): provides, nurtures, and guides. In this chapter, I am going to help you find your own personal 'guide'. This 'guide' will 'nurture' you if he is willing, as well as provide further guidance in your life.

Therefore, the first thing I want you to do – and you need to do - as you continue in this book is to find a 'substitute' for your father. I put 'substitute' in quotes because there is no perfect man who can replace your father: the one God intended you to have, but it didn't turn out that way. No man is ever going to care for you the way a God-fearing, natural father should and does care for his own son. But don't let this cause you unnecessary discouragement. There are many adult men out there who are willing and able to help you get through these rough and tumble teenage years with their advice and assistance. Your grandfather (if he is still with you), a sports coach, a teacher, a police officer you may know or sometimes come into contact with, the basketball referee at the local Boys & Girls Club, a Big Brother from the Big Brothers/Big Sisters organization (highly recommended!), even a member of the clergy, such as a priest or pastor from the church down the street – these are some possibilities of a 'substitute' father for you. Many adult men strive to make a better world, and that includes mentoring and guarding youth such as you. They are there, waiting with open arms for you. You must find them. At least one you must find and be open to.

It really doesn't matter which type of man-figure you find to help you and mentor you now as much as it is important that you do find an older man to help you and mentor you. Your mother whom you love more than anything cannot raise you to be a man. It cannot happen because it's impossible, and it puts your mother in a position she was never meant to be in. Nor can you raise yourself to be a man. Trying to do so on your own will lead to a dramatic and irreversible failure that will discourage you further and bring you way down low for good. Thus, it is a fact, you need right now some older man as an outside objective influence to be there to talk with you, walk with you, guide you, and help you with all your questions, problems, and issues you have, and are going to have, over the next several difficult years of your life. Going it alone just will not work, I'm sorry to say. I repeat: it will not work, no matter how hard you try or how good your own intentions for yourself are. You are definitely going to need an older man's influence and guidance as a mentor. All older men were once teenagers like you, so they have lived the experience already. Learn from one or more of them. It is the one best thing you can do to change and improve your situation right now.

Starting off with choosing a mentor, there are two things you must understand well. One, your mentor is not responsible for you in any way. That means he is not going to be the one who provides and meets your physical needs (food, clothing, shelter) for you, as your real father could have and should have. Real fathers provide for their children just as God intended. You yourself can make a promise right now that you will provide the needs someday if you have your own children. And if you do have children someday (I must admit, it is one of the greatest experiences in life to have your own children, as long as you are old enough, mature enough, and can provide for them.), hold yourself diligently to that promise you just made.

Second, don't expect perfection from any man of any age, because in some way every person on earth will disappoint you. If you reject anyone along the way of life's long journey for being imperfect, you will end up spending your life alone. The world is imperfect. People are imperfect. But don't let this discourage you in your search for a mentor. If you get tired and frustrated because you realize that your mentor is an imperfect person, and you realize that other people around you are imperfect, including you yourself, then you should be comforted by the fact that you have achieved a big step in normal, mature, rational reasoning, even without your natural father to help you with that understanding.

Communication will be the foundation of your relationship with your mentor. Whenever you meet with your mentor, look him eye-to-eye and smile and mean it. You can be nervous, that is okay. Just don't get overwhelmed with being nervous. Your mentor is there in that conversation for you because he wants to help you with whatever your issues are. Let that confidence settle your nervous stomach. One thing you can talk about is this book. Show him you are interested in the ideas in this book and see what he has to say.

Ask your mentor questions. Lots of questions. Never stop asking him, and anyone else you meet in your journey through life, many questions. Curiosity does not and did not 'kill the cat'. There is no such thing as a dumb question. The only dumb question is the one not asked. What is it you want to know right now that your mentor can answer for you? What about life is confusing for you that he can try and straighten out your understanding about it? Where can he assist you in your daily routines, or in life's various challenges, both simple and complex?

Listen to what he says, adjust your life, press on, listen to him again, adjust again, press on, go back and do it over again if necessary. A mentor is worth his weight in gold if he presses on with you and walks the distance with you faithfully to help you to get to where you want to go, from here to there, step by very small step.

Your mentor may become your best friend. It is one of the joys in life to have a best friend – someone close to you with whom you can share any idea, feeling, or hurt. You will have many male acquaintances and good friends you go to school with, or men you will someday work with, but most likely you will develop just a small number of 'best friends' in your life. Now, those best friends will be special for you, and can be with you all your life if you are lucky and work at the relationship but remember: they are only human and imperfect like you are. They have limitations in many areas of their own lives, just as you do. At times even a best friend will let you down, either intentionally or unintentionally. It doesn't matter if it was intentional or not: you must forgive them and your mentor when they do and move on to build up the relationship again. At the same time, I cannot stress this enough: be wary of anyone dangerous or badly influential to yourself.

In general, treat your mentor, your friends, and every man (and every woman) you encounter with respect and trust as long as it is warranted. You will be well served if you follow the bible's teachings here: treat others as you want to be treated yourself. Be at peace with your mentor and all mankind. When there are conflicts or problems with your mentor, try to work them out together if you can. This is a sign of maturity on your part. If he is a good man, he will be open to working out the issues between you.

This is important when interacting with a mentor: protect yourself. Only after you see consistent or dangerous problems with someone should you put up your guard. If your mentor gets too close to you physically, or makes you feel uncomfortable physically in any way, get away from him immediately any way you can. If you think it is entirely warranted, report him to the authorities immediately. Most men will not do harm to you physically or emotionally, but it still happens far too often in this cold, dark world we live in. Some men will prey on your trust, so you need to keep a sharp look out for wolves in sheep's clothing. This can be said also for 'friends' around you.

One last thing about your mentor: show him he is special to you. For example, after the first time you formally meet up with him, sit and write (not text message, not email, not typed, I mean write by your hand) a note to him saying 'thank you' and mean it, and then mail it to him. This will do a world of wonder for your relationship with him because it will show him that you are mature and ready for improvement and change with his help, and that you respect him as a man. After each and every time you meet with him, shake his hand and thank him for his time. If you exchange emails, text messages, or phone calls, always thank him for taking the time he took to respond to you and being involved in your life. It's all about communication and respect.

Chapter III - The Voice Inside

Here is a secret I wish I had learned at your age: No one will believe in you unless you first believe in yourself. That's a strong and very harsh reality in life. So, let me tell you right here, right now, little brother…**You have 'what it takes' to get through life and become a real man and be successful**. Your life will have meaning and a defined purpose. No matter how incompetent you feel at this very moment (and I felt incompetent for the first 34 years of my life, so I know well that there is great hope for you, my son.), you are not incomplete, you are not doomed to failure, and you can believe and trust in that little voice inside of you.

I can't do it! It's impossible! I so totally suck!

Is that what the little voice inside of you says? Those words (which are just a few of the many examples of the bold negatives you can and will tell yourself in your lifetime) are what Zig Ziglar, a famous motivational speaker during the 1970s and 1980s, called 'stinking-thinking'. Pay attention: you must avoid and crush stinking thinking with all your mind's strength to maintain a healthy self-image, strong self-confidence, and wholesome respect for yourself. This is very important for your personal development.

You will soon read in another chapter that your mind is like a trap that locks onto many outside influences. What you think in your heart is affected by what you put in your mind. And it works the same for your conscience – your 'gut instinct' – that God has given you as a human being separate from the animals. Why is this important to know? Because your actions will, without a doubt, follow your thoughts.

What your father would say or wouldn't say to you right now (if he were here) has so much importance that it would echo and magnify in your ears affecting you for a lifetime. Words have power. The bible says that the tongue has the power to build up and the power to destroy. Sticks and stones may break some bones, but words can break a heart. You already know that if you have ever been cruelly bullied. You need strong encouragement, and this is where the mentor comes into place. He will be the one who encourages you after that basketball game loss, or the low-grade on the Spanish quiz, or being rejected by the girl you developed a crush on. Coming back from a loss is always hard, but it is never impossible. With good encouragement from your mentor and positive thoughts on your own part, you can overcome any harsh loss.

It goes even deeper than that. Much deeper. Deeper inside your heart and soul.

Just once, I am sure, you would give anything just to hear: "I am proud of you, I believe in you, I am in your corner, you have what it takes, and I love you!" Not hearing those phrases may make you believe inside that you are a boy to be ashamed of, flawed, unacceptable, unlovable and unloved. And maybe you might feel that, if your father were around to give you the least bit of encouragement, you would turn into some entitled and spoiled brat. This is so not true! It would have made a world of positive difference if your father were around to encourage you. But possibly after reading this book you won't waste decades of your life (like I unfortunately did) finally figuring out that you are not so bad after all. Many men go through their entire lives wondering what happened to them to make them end up a 'broken loser'. Often times it was their own fault because of their own actions both as a child and as an adult. So, for you, it all begins with the correct and positive thinking about yourself, and then the choices and actions you can make corresponding to the age you are now at and will be at in the future. Just by reading this book right now you are showing yourself that you care about yourself and you want a better, improved life for yourself. That is a great start, little brother! Your father isn't here to give you this encouraging start in life, so you must find it for yourself. As you will see everywhere in this book, thinking positively and purely about yourself has so many good benefits.

You might say to yourself, "I'll be happy when...". When what? When you get those new Air Jordan kicks? When you have a million dollars in the bank? When you get your first BMW sports car? When you have sex for the first time? As you will see in a later chapter, happiness with these worldly lusts is temporary and ultimately so very unfulfilling. True happiness comes from knowing 'The Secret' in your heart. (Go on and look ahead at the chapter "Keeping It Real" if you are intrigued now with this concept.)

Your attitude counts most of all as it affects all your actions. Change is seldom easy, but it is far from being impossible, and your attitude about change makes all the difference. You must believe that you can change, and when you believe that you can do it, you will do it. Everything begins with your thinking positively. From your thoughts are born your actions: be they your virtues or your vices. God gave you as a human being the ability to think and reason, unlike the rest of His Creation. As such, God does not want you to make the wrong choices in life. Think things through carefully and thoroughly and make the right choices (you will see this theme a lot in this book). Difficulties and challenges in life can make you better…or bitter. The choice is yours to make what you want with what you have been given or sit on the couch and pout about "being screwed over in life".

Think positively about yourself and others, and you will act accordingly. If you are constantly putting yourself down, or putting other people down, such as being a bully to the weak kid in the class, you are never going to respect yourself or gain respect in society. Bad thinking and wrong actions only bring you way down, and once you start on the road of forever negativity, it is very difficult to stop and bring yourself back up. For example, being a jerk leads to big problems and then even bigger problems when dealing with other people. Even if no other people are directly involved, your actions affect yourself. Stealing a candy bar from the local convenience store will lead you to one day stealing a liquor bottle from the corner liquor store, and then increasingly cause you to reach 'higher' (which is actually really reaching 'lower') to fulfill your ever-demanding lusts with more bad actions, such as then stealing a car from your neighbor down the block.

Doing bad things to other people and bad-mouthing other people are like a drug, because sin such as vengeance is pleasurable to the flesh. You know this already, I am sure. You can become addicted to negative talk and bad actions just as if they were an illegal drug. Look at the strange newspapers in the supermarket checkout lanes. Aren't the stories all about tearing people down, not building them up? (Negativity sells this trash.) And if you do develop an addiction to treating people wrongly, breaking that addiction is paramount to improving your life to refocus on a better direction. Otherwise you will suffer consequences you won't like, such as end up in jail, or worse, dead. Respect yourself by respecting others around you. It is the only way to live correctly in a civilized society, even if everything and everyone else around you is failing you and falling apart at the seams.

The same goes true with respecting authority. If you reject proper authority, then you come off as being a jerk in the world, and no one worth anything in life will ever respect you in return. At the same time, however, you need to weigh advice from authority (and your mentor as well) carefully, because very often people have 'agendas'. Their 'agendas' may not line up with yours, and they will even - purposely or not - steer you wrong. Some kinds of people may indeed be selfish and seek only what is best for themselves first and put your needs, wants, and desires second, but thankfully these people are rare in the world. If you happen to come across such misaligned people in authority and they do not help you, get away from them as you are able to, for this situation will only get you further frustrated at the world. Being frustrated, you will be unable to accomplish anything because you need the help of good people in authority in order to get ahead. Your mother, the police, the judge (if you go before one), the school principal, and other people in authority are usually looking out for your best interests, but, again I will repeat it, that is not always the case. If, also, you do not assess the influence of an authority figure adequately, you will be surpassed and stepped on by all the jerks of the world who do not give a flip about that authority. These people who disrespect authority you will be able to see and figure out easily and interacting with them will only cause unnecessary problems for you. Avoid these jerks. Furthermore, if you are careful on how you follow the advice and instructions of authority – go with your gut, believe your conscience, it is rarely wrong - you will sleep better at night and have an easier time in the world. It's a balancing act.

All institutions and all people will want you to believe in them and follow them because that is how they grow and maintain themselves. But be wise. Even though they are inviting and appear wholesome, not all of them are good or beneficial for you. You are going to have to be discerning about which ones to follow. No one can make those decisions of discernment for you. A person can get along with institutions and people and still disagree with them, if necessary. That is a great sign of a real, mature man. Be loyal to all your relationships with the right people and institutions, but never disregard your own conscience, your gut instinct. Your personal growth and self-reliance will require you to rely on Your Creator who gave you this gut instinct versus the other people who will entice you or pull you into their issues.

Believe in that small voice – your gut instinct - inside of you. Treasure it and grow with it. It is yours and yours alone. Don't agree to what is just good or just better but agree to what is truly and really the best. This will take steady and continuing discipline on your part, and again no one can make those decisions for you. If you always look to others to make the hard decisions for you, then you will fail miserably, no questions asked. You must make up your mind and your heart by yourself to do what is right and follow the truth.

Discernment is not an opinion or a rash judgment. Opinions and beliefs have more destructive power than any weapons in the world, as many people are led astray by those who intentionally do evil. Believe it because it happens all too often in this world. Trust the gut instinct the Good Lord put in your heart. There will be much false discernment from the world placed before you trying to lead you far astray from what is good and true. There will be many enticing voices and many tempting attractions in your life trying to take you off the 'Correct Path' for your life's journey. Your compass to stay on track is your conscience, your discernment, your gut instinct, that little voice inside of you. Don't let yourself get off the track of following what is right and true. Never, ever. If you do, you will be saddened quickly, feel guilty, and if you are off the track long enough, you will fall into a deep depression. Don't let his happen to you. Listen to that still, small voice inside of you for all your decisions and directions. It wants what is best for you.

Chapter IV - Your Reputation

"To this above all else, to thine own self be true, and then as night follows the day, thou can do no wrong." – William Shakespeare

Do you want people to stop saying you are stupid? Then stop doing stupid things!

What is this 'stupid thing' you are talking about?

It's quite simple. Let's quote Forrest Gump (from the movie) on what a stupid thing is, "Mama always said 'Stupid is as stupid does'." Yes, it's true my friend, if you do a stupid thing, then others will think you are stupid. They will also think you will continue to do stupid things, and they will thus ignore you. Little brother trust me on this, because I learned this lesson the hard way, from my life experience. The great American actor John Wayne also said it best, "Life is tough. It's even tougher if you're stupid."

But that decision not to do stupid things is entirely up to YOU and your choices that you make in life (there's that word again: choices). The bible says (and I am paraphrasing here) that even if you give a fool a hundred years to change, he will still always be a fool. Don't be like this! Look to change your thoughts and actions today away from stupidity! Your reputation depends on it.

But what if I don't think what I'm doing is stupid? What then?

If ten-million-and-one people do a stupid thing, then it is still a stupid thing. No doubts about it. For example, people all over the world use vulgar language. You probably hear it every day. Doesn't it make the person speaking that way sound stupid and ignorant?

As I write this chapter, just a few days ago a college student, who had been sentenced to fifteen years hard labor in a North Korean prison, was flown back to the USA in a coma, and soon after died. He had originally been caught at North Korea's airport customs with a stolen poster when he was about to leave the country. Now, people can argue with each other until they are blue in the face whether or not this young man was stupid to go to North Korea in the first place. (My take is, yes, he was stupid to go to such a violent country, whose leader will have you executed if you look at him cross-eyed). But certainly, it is without a doubt STUPID that he first entered a place he was not supposed to go (the restricted area of the hotel he was staying in) and then stole something that didn't belong to him (the propaganda poster 'as a souvenir'). Stupid! And, another recent college graduate from the USA was partying on a Greek Island in a bar at 3am (3am? Yes. He should have been asleep in his hotel room, no?), and got into a fight that turned into a 9-on-1 street brawl. He ended up dead as well. Stupid!

Do you see how stupid actions can be have irreversible and serious consequences?

We make hundreds of decisions each and every day, some small, and most not noticeable to others. But some have far reaching consequences that affect our own futures and the lives of those around us deeply. You have a choice with these decisions: Are you going to do the right thing, or the wrong (stupid) thing?

Yes, right now you are underage (a 'minor'), and you are subject to many 'authorities' who can, must, and will make many decisions for you, with or without your consent. It doesn't matter much what you have to say in such circumstances. You have to take what is presented to you and required of you. Such authorities may be your mother (or other guardians), your school teachers, the school principal, and even, if you get into serious enough trouble, police officers and judges. Part of being young means you are not ready yet for adult decisions. At the same time, no one should expect you to make adult decisions right now. You are just a kid, and believe me, that is okay. Really. Stay a kid and enjoy being a kid. But even though you are not making adult decisions, you still make countless decisions daily which affect you now and will affect you in the future in many ways. For example:

Are you going to finish that homework assignment due tomorrow? Or just get a failing grade?

Are you going to listen to your mother telling you to do the dishes and take out the trash? Or will you blow her off and disrespect her?

Are you going to get yourself 'too involved' with that pretty girl you are interested in, and then, as a complete mistake that you had no intention of doing, get her pregnant?

Are you going to join the gang at the street corner? (You know who I am talking about: the homeboys who sell drugs and steal from convenience stores, and who may even carry weapons.)

This of course is just a very small list of sample decisions you must face every day in your life. Some of these are more serious situations you must face, I agree, but there will be others in your life until your last breath that you must face. The decisions you make now will have lasting effects on yourself, others around you, and possibly even your own wife and children someday.

But all my 'friends' are doing it (whatever bad decision 'it' is)? Why can't I?

The bible says not to pay attention to those others around you (Even if they are your friends. Maybe they shouldn't be.) who are doing wrong things. Why? Because those people "have no future". That's what it says in Proverbs. It makes no sense to do actions that are bad and evil, because, if you seriously think about it, you are only leading yourself downhill to your own destruction. You will make mistakes in life, everyone does. There is no shame in making honest mistakes. And there will be regrets, too. Oh, so many of them. There isn't a human that has ever lived that didn't have some regrets. And yes, you ARE a sinner. That is unavoidable, as your bad thoughts and omissions of doing good are enough to label you a sinner. Some of those seemingly innocent 'mistakes' you will make are really going to end up being pretty serious. There is absolutely no good reason, none, to go down the road to destruction by doing evil. There is nothing to be gained – that's all an illusion that the darkness in this world wants you to believe is good for you. You may not be popular for doing the right thing and avoiding the wrong thing but doing the right thing will always win out in the end. It always has, and it always will. Always.

You can be sure that you will always be better off avoiding stupidity. As one very famous - and hot! - actress once said in a popular 1990s television advertisement, "Being smart is sexier than being stupid any day".

Chapter V – Achieving Success

Success means accomplishing a goal. Goal setting begins with seeing what you want in life. Can you honestly say that you are really ready to leave the past behind and move forward?

Life is fluid and ever-evolving. Changes can happen for you if you want them to. No one can make the changes you want. You have to do it yourself. And as was said in a previous chapter: if you don't believe in yourself, don't expect anyone else to believe in you.

A wonderfully fantastic man I once knew, a mentor of mine named Roy Cook (may he rest in peace), told me that "If you don't know where you are going, you are sure to get there.". This is true of all of life, and it is especially true in the importance of setting goals. Do you ever think about where you want to be when you are in your late teens (just to start), early 20s (thinking bigger!), or even later? Can you easily clarify what it is you want in life? How about what you want just for this year, this month, this week, or just by the end of today?

If you want to achieve success in life you need to set some *goals*. All of your focus in life will be either on your goals or off your goals. There is no other direction that your focus will go. You need to be conscious over all of your own efforts and abilities. No one else can do it for you, even though others may, and hopefully will, help you along the way. Goals have to be consciously made, and they must have accountability. If you have found a trustworthy older man who can keep you accountable to your goals, then that makes you half-way towards a successful celebration because you are able to communicate what it is that you want to achieve.

Think about your goals clearly. If you say in your mind "I want to have $2,000 in the bank by the time I am 18", that is a goal that you have defined, can now communicate to someone else (such as your mentor), and can surely achieve if you put in the right efforts. But if you just say, "I want to be rich", that isn't a good goal because it isn't defined enough. Without definition, a goal will never be realized. You need to consider many things when setting goals, including the time and resources and abilities available to you to reach success. Your goals in life will always take effort, and that effort has to come from inside of you alone. A mentor can encourage you, but your goals are yours alone to pursue and no one else will work them out for you. Let me repeat that another way: *no one else will do for you what you need to do for yourself.*

This leads to an important point about setting goals. A goal must be something that you are passionate about. If it doesn't really interest you, then you won't put much effort into it, and then you are likely to fail. Failure often leads to discouragement which leads to more failures and the cycle goes round and round. What do you love? What is truly important for you? As the bible says, "Where your treasure is, there your heart will be". The priorities you have will be a big determinant in the goals you set for yourself.

Again, you need to be able to communicate to another person what your goals are. It can help to just get a sheet of paper and a pencil (better than a pen, you can erase and adjust) and just start brainstorming: *What is it I want in life?* Once you have a good and worthy list, and checked it over several times, go to your mentor and sit and talk with him about your goals. If he takes the time to be with you and discuss your goals, then take good advantage of that availability and any advice he gives to you. It is truly precious that someone else takes an interest in our goals. Don't forget to ask him questions about your goals you need help with. Also, what does he think about your goals? Is there anyone else he recommends you talk about your goals with? The bible says that "there is wisdom in the counsel of many". This means that the more men you have advising you on your goals and goal setting, the better your perspective will be on them, and the more you will learn about yourself and your own limitations. Learn as you communicate with others and you will advance in life faster than you can imagine.

You can't just say you wish for something and expect it to happen. Life doesn't work that way. Goals are what made billionaires rich, professional athletes stars, and rock musicians' celebrities. But they didn't start off saying they were going to be billionaires, or professional athletes, or big rock stars. They all began small and built their lives one small step at a time. How do you eat an elephant? One bite at a time. (And you start at the right end!)

Goals must start off small and few, and then get bigger and more numerous over time. Start off with a micro-goal, something you can define and accomplish in the immediate. You cannot say, "I want to be a millionaire!" or "I want to travel all over Europe!" and expect it to happen soon. Unless you manage to create the next greatest app for the iPhone, the chances of you becoming a millionaire anytime soon are zero. And making it to Europe has to start with many other small (micro) goals, such as getting a birth certificate to help you apply for a passport and accumulating enough funds to support yourself during your trip. Instead, try "I want to have $3,000 in the bank by the time I am 18. This money will be used for educational purposes or travelling to Europe". In that way, you have defined a small goal that can be reached ("$3000 by 18 years old"), and you are able to tell someone else why the goal is important for you ("for educational purposes or travelling to Europe"). The timeline is up to you, as is the size of the goal, but please be reasonable and patient with yourself. Remember: you are just a kid right now, and no one should expect you to be able to follow adult level responsibilities (goals) yet for a very long time. Start off with a few small goals you can reach this week, and then this month, and see where that takes you. A snowball rolls and gets bigger as it continues rolling on and on. It's the same with goals.

As your goals get bigger, they must take you to a point of success within the time-frames you have set. With the bad example above ("I want to be a millionaire!") there is no time-frame and thus no chance of it happening. At the same time, you don't want to set goals that are too easy to achieve and don't create challenges for you. "I want to make $20 before the end of the month." Yeah, you could probably do that by the end of today (if you are really ready to work), but how does that lead you to bigger and better goals? There is little challenge to develop you in any way.

Your time-frame must be reasonable, but it also must have an element of 'urgency'. This will help you focus and keep yourself on track to achieve your goals. This does not mean that you go wild and work on your goal for 48 hours straight without sleep. You still have your personal life to manage and taking care of yourself is *a long-term goal in itself.* A key part of this is making an action-plan. What do you need to do to accomplish your goal? What resources do you need? How do you start off? Is assistance from someone else needed? How much time per day, per week, per month will you put into it without depriving yourself in other areas of your life? Writing down this action-plan and then discussing it with your mentor will help you in achieving your goals.

Okay, you have read a lot about goals so far. Let's try something. Here is a quick exercise I want you to try right now: get a blank piece of paper and a marker or pen, and DRAW what you want to accomplish in the next year (trust me on this, it might seem difficult, but we are starting small here). It doesn't matter if you are a Monet artist or you suck with crayons. The point is that you can VISUALIZE on paper what it is you want out of life for the next year. This drawing will help you 1. See the goal, 2. Believe in the goal, and 3. Do the actions necessary towards the goal. After you finish the drawing, show it to someone you respect, like your mother, a teacher, or your mentor. That, there, is being able to communicate your goal, which we already know from reading this chapter is a key step in accomplishing your goal.

So, here's the end of the chapter on goals. I will ask you, little brother: what is your goal for today? If you said, "To finish reading this book", then I would say that is not a good goal. Yes, finishing reading this book is a good idea to accomplish at some point, but the information in this book is thick and must be slowly digested. Reading it all at once will only cause you to forget key ideas. It's important to follow your goals with 'baby steps'. You have finished this chapter now. Did you draw the picture of your goal for the upcoming year (from the above paragraph)? If you did, then that was one micro-goal for today that you can pursue further. What is another goal you can achieve today?

Chapter VI – Dealing with Failure

Fear will probably be your biggest obstacle in all that you want to do. Facing your fear while being responsible for yourself and relying on no one else is the greatest good you can do for yourself. This will also be very important for your own family someday. You will become a true, honorable man this way. That ideal doesn't come from getting older and bigger. It takes more than physically growing and aging. Through your successes and failures, you will learn, mature, and become a man.

Life requires constant action. Put strong efforts and diligence into your actions and your life will reward you greatly in return. If you choose to be lazy and blow off important actions you need to be doing, you will in the end lose out on many of life's greatest rewards.

The good idea: You are a unique, special individual, and you have much in yourself to offer the world, and the world has much available to offer you in return.

The good reality: God brought you to it ('some difficulty'), and He will bring you through it.

There will be challenges in front of you always and everywhere. Even just getting ahead in life involves you doing something you have a passion for because then you will tend to do it well. Do you know yourself to be talented in something? You will still need to put a lot of effort into it if you want to make a big career of it. There is a lot of solid competition out there, and unlike in the old days when you just competed against someone else in your town or city, now you are literally competing against people from around the world.

It is important to be engaged in something on a regular basis that makes you feel a little bit special. You need something that sets you apart from others. Some people like to draw. Some play a musical instrument. Others (like me) like to write. Hobbies are good, and sometimes a hobby can develop into a paying career (if you are lucky). Maybe there are several things you can do, but whatever they are, they must make you feel successful in life. Success helps keep you excited about life and help you experience the good life more.

Success in life is not necessarily dependent on fame, glory, or riches like we think when we are younger and immature. Success is about meaning in life (which you will read a lot about in a later chapter). Yes, if you have a meaningful life you will be satisfied. What is meaningful to you? Often meaning comes from helping others. Or, it can come when you struggle to do something that is challenging and finally accomplish it. It is true that you have to be always working at something to be truly happy. The quick and easy life is never beneficial, no matter how tempting it is. Hollywood, the music business, and professional sports are full of celebrities who do damaging and self-destructive things to themselves because they are not truly happy with their lives as they live them.

When dealing with the world: Make it your own. At least within and around yourself, establish a place where you can deal with problems and issues on your own agenda and timeline. Some people call it a "man cave". It's a place or a state of mind where you can tune out and take a breather. The world is a challenging place that seems impossible to handle at times. Allow yourself to recuperate from time to time, and you can come out stronger and deal with life and its issues better.

Of course, a lot of life is just routine. This is just taking care of yourself. Conversely, a lot of life is just plain fun as you allow yourself to be who you are. Woody Allen, an older comic actor, said in one of his earlier films, that "95% of life is just showing up". So true that is! There are times when it's tough and you want to quit whatever it is you are doing. But then the thing to remember is that the situation can always get better for you in many ways. Always.

Can you rise to the top? I think you can, but it will take time. Malcolm Gladwell, a world-famous sociologist, said it takes 10,000 hours of practice to become an expert in one single activity. 10,000 hours! That means if you want to be a great soccer goalie, you will stand in front of a soccer goal with others taking hard shots on you for 10,000 hours. During those 10,000 hours, there will be wins, and there will be losses. Deal with both accordingly. Can you be a gracious winner and be thankful to the opponent(s) for challenging you? Can you accept loss without losing your own pride and getting discouraged? It's your attitude during that 10,000 hours of practice that matters most.

Another example close to my heart: if you want to be a great author (like I am trying to be with the fiction novels I write), then you are going to have to sit in front of a computer screen and type away for 10,000 hours until you create that perfect piece of literature. Now, of course it is impossible to accomplish 10,000 hours of writing - or 10,000 hours of anything - in a one, two, or even five-year time-frame. You are going to need at least a decade to accomplish the 10,000 hours of that single activity you want to be an expert at. The advantage that you have, little brother, is that you are still young. You hopefully have decades upon decades ahead of you in life. Becoming an expert on something close and dear to your heart is well within your reach. You just have to have the self-discipline and self-motivation to go for it!

What do you need to ensure you achieve success? You need 1. A good, healthy self-image of yourself, 2. Perseverance to never quit even when it seems impossible that you will be successful, and 3. Positive feedback from someone you trust. The combination of these three elements will not guarantee that you will be successful, but the chances are much greater than trying without them. And what if you are not seeing success at what you are attempting? Step-back. Re-evaluate. Make the necessary changes. Take another step forward. It really is that easy.

No one can predict the future. The unexpected is always around the corner. Errors and mistakes are for sure going to be an unavoidable part of your life. Remember this: you have every right to make mistakes. No one likes to admit that they made a mistake, but you must admit your mistakes if you want to mature and grow. Have the courage to take ownership of the mistakes you commit. Learn the value of humility in admitting you made a mistake. You can always bounce back from any mistake you make, no matter how big it is. Perhaps your mistake came from irrational thinking, how can you change this behavior? Just don't rely on your emotions to make your behavioral changes. Prepare yourself as best as you can to accept failures, and as you learn from your mistakes, you will save yourself a lot of heartache later. Don't overestimate yourself in anything or you will most likely lead yourself to failure. Of course, the opposite is true: don't underestimate your own skills, abilities, and experiences which can carry you through difficult and challenging times. Moreover, do not pay attention to negative talk from anyone concerning your failures and mistakes. Keeping your mind free of negativity will help you avoid making mistakes in the future.

If what you did was *wrong* and rather than just an honest mistake, be prepared to deal with the consequences from your school, your mother/guardian, or even the law. *Sinful acts* will harm your soul. The guilt you will feel from committing sins is painful, but it is healthy. Ask God to forgive you each and every time. Similarly, hurting others requires you to say you are sorry and ask them for forgiveness. Follow this up by confessing what you did wrong to your mentor or a member of the clergy in order to keep yourself humble. Talk about it with them. How can you keep from doing these wrongful acts again? Mature people find answers to that question daily.

Often times your failure is not totally your fault. People are going to let you down, put you down, and even leave you to fail without them helping you. That's an undeniable and unfortunate fact of life when dealing with an imperfect society. Forgive people who wrong you each and every time, no matter how grave the offense is, and move on from there. There is nothing to be gained from dwelling and stewing on a failure that someone else caused for you. You will not 'win' by holding onto that position of unforgiveness. That does not mean you forget the offense or that you must continue to associate with that person. But forgiving others is a big step in personal growth. Start doing it while you are young, and it will be easier when you are older. This includes forgiving yourself for your inadequacies and the many mistakes you make. Forgive, and move on, my friend. You will feel better about yourself and your life if you do.

Chapter VII - Work

Work can be defined as *helping other* people. Take that idea further and we see that *you can get what you want when you help other people get what they want*. Work is difficult and tiring, but it is part of the human condition that we need to work. Your first work right now is your schooling. Don't let anyone tell you that school is not work. Do it diligently and as best as you can. In addition to doing school-work, *working a job* has rewards. If you are under 16 years old, the government says you are too young to work a formal job. But there are still ways you can earn money by working: raking leaves and shoveling snow for an elderly neighbor, or even walking a dog. Your ability to work is not hindered by your age. When you start out young, you should take whatever job you can get. You can be proud of yourself for this work and be very happy to have some money in your pocket. You might even feel a little rich. But be aware of it now: the world, and North America especially, demands great sums of money for even an ordinary adult life. In the long run as an adult, you will need a fairly good paying job. Only bad guys need to read this part: selling drugs and other crimes may pay well in dollars, but these "jobs" always inevitably end up getting you thrown in prison and/or killed. Sooner or later the choice to be criminal squashes you flat. You really don't want to go that way, little brother. Be legitimate and true to yourself and society in your work. It's the only way to go.

Everyone needs formal education or training to get a decent paying adult job. There is no way around that fact. Low skills pay low wages. And let's get real here: even if you like to play the guitar, the chances are you are not going to be the next John Lennon or Kurt Cobain. Even if you play football well at the high school level, the chances are you are not going to be on the Redskins roster someday. This is part of the goal setting chapter you read earlier: you want to be practical in picking what field of work you will do and start to prepare for it as soon as you are able. I know a young man who has been playing the guitar since he was nine years old. He plays the bass and guitar extremely well and is hired out by different bands when they need him. He has his own band. He has made a fantastic CD of his own creative music. But he still has his "day job" to pay the big bills in life. He sells smartphones. He would be flat broke if he did not have this real daytime job.

Highly skilled jobs will almost always require a college education or formal training. Talk with your mentor about your thoughts for a career. Also, go to your career counseling department at your high school and see how they can help you. This is an invaluable resource that you are lucky to have, but many kids blow will just off. The more you discuss your plans, the better informed you will be to make decisions about your future.

College is brutally expensive in North America. By getting scholarships for good grades or good athletic abilities (primarily, but it is not limited to these two characteristics), you can achieve your college dreams. As soon as you can in your junior year of high school, start looking into scholarships through online websites. There are a myriad of scholarships available, and not just merit based. There is even a scholarship you can apply for by just being left-handed! You can also make college cheaper by joining the military and getting the G.I. Bill. Also, you can go to a local Community College for two years, which is a lot less expensive than a state or private university, and then transfer. I know of one student who did exceptionally well at an unknown Community College in his town for two years and then transferred with a full-ride to Harvard University. That is something you can aspire to! Not all of us are Einstein or Tom Brady or Bill Gates, but we can find what we are good at during our education experiences and focus on that. Pick what you think you will like which also can provide a solid living. It used to be that a college degree in anything would set you up for life. A degree in literature or sociology at one time got you a job easily. Now, the situation is you have to aim better than that. Focus on what the world will need by the time you graduate.

Not every boy needs to go to college to be successful. There are perfectly good and well-paid careers in the trades: plumbing, welding, electrical, auto mechanics (to name a few). For a trade, you will still need some kind of formal advanced training from other men who are already professionals, though. So, yeah, get that advanced certificate or license or degree that is necessary, and you can start making some real money. It's almost certain you will have to start on the ground floor, but at least you can work your way up.

As for being hopeful that someday you will be a Youtuber or actor or a musical wonder on the world's stages, there is still much you need to understand here. Don't make a big effort about trying to emulate their accomplishments in the working world. They cannot be a mentor or role model to you if they don't know you. Watching a celebrity on a screen will not help you learn much about life. Do you find them entertaining? Then ok, enjoy them as entertainers. But don't for a minute believe that means their lives should be emulated by you. Every generation has popular people, sports heroes, music celebrities and movie stars who have made it big in life with fame and fortune, but they are few in number. Reality is much different. You aren't going to suddenly be a rap star and you aren't suddenly going to be picked to win the actor-lottery. In reality, it must be a terribly difficult job for many of these famous people because so many end up with tragic personal lives. Oftentimes their lives are ruined and shortened by the serious, irreversible mistakes they make as celebrities. There are too many statistics supporting that statement throughout history to say it has no merit.

So, get an education in something the world needs, and earn a decent and honest living to support yourself. Then, when you have your family, you can support them, too. Support means costs, but it also means saving. Whenever you get a paycheck, put aside some of that money. Save as much as you are able to. Life will always make unexpected financial demands of you. The car you own will need repair, or your paid-for smartphone will get lost. There is always something coming around the corner you didn't expect, so don't blow your whole Friday paycheck on a weekend of fun. Save for these emergencies. If you don't, you will eventually have no choice but to be borrowing from others or using credit cards. In a very quick while you will be in dire financial straits that are almost impossible to get out of. Dave Ramsey, a famous money guru on the radio and in financial self-help books, says that everyone should start out with $1,000 in an emergency fund. You may be too young to achieve this amount right now, but as you get older and your bills get bigger, putting aside for emergencies will be of significant importance. Don't put it off or you will never do it. A little bit held for the unexpected will save a whole heap of problems later on.

I am of age now, but I don't know how to get a job! Who would ever want to hire me?

This is more of the 'stinking thinking' that you need to stop in your mind. You can get the job, my friend, but it is going to take some good effort on your part. The job is not going to come to your front door looking for you. You are going to have to go after it. Research the many places to work at which are looking for new employees. Look online for their websites and any recent news about the companies to help you learn about what they do and the jobs they offer. Mail (or fill out online) applications to all the places you want to work at. Don't think now about where it is best for you to work at, whether it is worthwhile to send an application to someplace or not. That final decision is best made AFTER you have received all the formal offers for the jobs you applied for. If you don't have a resume, look up on the internet examples to use specific to the type of job you are applying for. Don't worry if you don't have much to place in the 'education' and 'experience' parts of your resume, as the person who will look at your resume already knows something about who you are and where you come from. The employer won't expect more from you than you can offer at that moment. If you need a cover letter to go with an application, again, look online for examples to use. Don't copy the cover letters you find online word for word. Tailor them to fit the job and your character. Also, get the name of someone specific in the Human Resources department or a manager to address the cover letter to. A cover letter that is addressed to no one in particular will find itself in the 'circular file' (that is, the trash can).

Next you need to prepare for the interview, if you are asked to come in for one. Research the company beforehand so you know information about the position you want and about the company itself. If you walk into the interview with no knowledge about how the company is run, what it does, or who owns it, you are not going to get the job. The day of the interview, shower, shave, and comb your hair. It is often said: Dress for Success. When you go for a job interview, dress your very best. Don't wear baggy pants/jeans and a t-shirt and Nike kicks. Goodwill and The Salvation Army have dress shirts, suits, shoes, and ties very cheap to buy. The Salvation Army even has a program that if you absolutely cannot afford to dress nicely for an upcoming interview, they will provide you with a suit, shirt, shoes and a tie at no cost. Take advantage of that program. If you have a tattoo, cover it up (if you can with clothing, but don't use makeup to do so if it is on your face or neck). If you have an earring or nose-ring, take it out. Don't wear any jewelry, not even a ring on your finger. You are making all this extra effort because you want to look responsible, mature, and up to the task of the job which you are applying for. When you meet the interviewer, offer your right hand for a firm handshake. Smile and mean it. Relax, he or she isn't going to shoot you down right then and there – you have been given a chance to meet the interviewer, and that shows the company is interested in you already! Don't slouch in your chair; sit up straight, legs uncrossed but together, and move your hands gently and formally as you speak. Don't speak over the interviewer. Listen carefully and answer all of the interviewer's questions accurately and honestly. If you don't know the answer to a question, say so, don't make up an answer or lie. Look the interviewer right in the eye when you answer a question. Impress the interviewer with questions about the company and position which you have memorized in advance. For example: ask what the job-skills requirements are. Ask who you will be working with. Ask how you can be valuable to the company in the long run. The more questions you ask, the more it shows that you are interested in working there. A moment of silence between you and the interview is not bad, but if you can, ask another question. The interview is over when the interviewer, not you, leads it to be over. When you stand up as the interview is over, be sure to tell the interviewer that you enjoyed meeting with him or her and that you are very interested in the position offered. After the interview, write (don't type) a 'thank you' note to the person who gave you the interview and mail it immediately. This will show your earnestness in wanting to get the job offered to you. It will also impress your interviewer greatly because few people do this anymore. If you are finally offered a position, don't put off for too long accepting (or denying, if there are other, better offers) the position because the person making the hiring decision is under a time-constraint and may not wait for you. Even if you don't accept the offer, respond graciously to the person making the hiring decision for the position you applied for, because, who knows? You may want to work there after all someday.

Once you have the job, get ready to show up early your first day, showered, shaven, and dressed appropriately. If you are going to be flipping burgers at McDonalds, no need to wear a suit and tie. If you are going to be in an office, jeans and Air Jordan kicks will make you look stupid and out of place. You might be nervous seeing all the new people around you. Be cheerful with each person you meet, especially your boss. As has been said, and it is still true, there is no second chance at making a good first impression. How you come across now will effectively set the way you will be treated at this company. Follow instructions for the work you will be doing and don't be afraid to ask questions if you don't know something. Your manager is there to guide you, so listen to him or her. Do the work quickly and efficiently, not wasting time or the company's resources. As you leave at the end of every workday, say goodbye to your boss with a smile.

Working a job is sometimes seen as an 'unfortunate' part of life. But I hope that as you get older, you will see the value that work can have in your own life, and how much value you can add to the world with your work. It gives a person's life lots of meaning and sustains us. So, be smart and get a job.

Chapter VIII – Money

This is one the longest chapters in the book because it is such an important topic that few people talk about openly. Yes, your friends are going to compare salaries and their wallets with one another and with you, but rarely do people talk about the best ways to save and manage their monies. This chapter will be an introduction to helping you do that.

You got your first paycheck. Pat yourself on the back for the good work you did and the money your honestly earned! You may even feel a little rich right now. Just don't go wild and blow through your Friday paycheck over the weekend. Many people say it religiously: *Pay yourself first*. Save a little each and every paycheck, no matter how little your savings is. This will help establish a habit right off that will serve you well all your life. Nothing is safer for your hard-earned money than a simple savings account in a bank or credit union, even with interest rates paying close to zero percent, as it is better than keeping it at home where it can become 'lost or stolen' or spent easily. Albert Einstein (possibly the greatest genius ever in human history, also mentioned somewhere else in this book) said that the greatest human invention is 'compound interest', where the money you put in a savings account earns interest after the first year, and then the second year interest is earned not just on the money you first put in but also on the interest accumulated at the end of the first year, and the same goes for the third year, and so on and so on. You can only win when you save. Even if you are only able to put a little bit away each paycheck into a savings account in a bank, you will be far ahead of all your peers in a few short years. The majority of North Americans do not save anything – not a single dollar. That is a really bad statistic you don't want to be a part of.

Plan and budget your money every month and every paycheck. Every dollar you earn should have a 'label' placed on it, telling you how it was earned and where it will go. Know how many dollars you earn in a month (for example) just as you know how you earned it and spend only what is planned/budgeted for. As every dollar is labeled, you can thereby save some of them rather than spend it all. This is called 'living below your means'. This new habit for you will reward you all of your life. If you can't live below your means, you will instead go into the habit of debt. To then go back to living below your means you, have only two choices: earn more and/or spend less. There are no other options here.

You have some money to save. Great, little brother, good job! Where do you put it now? Credit Unions are better to put your money into than banks, for many reasons. The first, and big reason, is that banks usually charge hefty fees for depositing money into them if you don't maintain a minimum balance. For example: one large national bank charges $12 per month if you don't keep $1,000 minimum in the bank. That, to me, is a pure scam. Why should you pay a bank when they lend your money to someone else and collect interest on it? Credit Unions do not charge these kinds of fees. Don't worry about your credit union not being big or national. Many Credit Unions have connections with one another, so you can go into most any credit union branch in the country and do your banking without any extra fees or having to have a local account. Credit Unions are also more forgiving if you bounce a check or overdraw your account (still, bad ideas anyway, don't do it). Banks will bleed you through the nose with bounced check and overdraft fees. Credit Unions are connected with ATM's just like banks, and very often can be fee-free as well if you use an ATM. If you do go with a bank (maybe it is close to your home), make sure you understand the fees, especially fees for taking money out of ATM's that are not 'in-network'. These ATM fees and other bank fees will quickly drain your account. Credit Unions also offer better interest rates for loans. This is good, for example when you are older, and you want to buy a car. While it is always better to pay cash for everything (except possibly a home), getting a Credit Union loan can make sense if you need a car to get to your job. No matter which you use, bank or a credit union, check to see if you can log into your accounts online. If you can, check your accounts online a few times a week to see how you are spending versus saving. Checking your accounts online frequently is also good to make sure that your identity hasn't been stolen or that someone isn't stealing from you.

Sometimes opening a savings account at a bank or credit union without a parent's/guardian's permission and co-signature is not possible until you are 18 years old. Maybe also you don't have a parent or guardian you can fully trust to be named on the account with you. If that is the unfortunate case for you, follow this excellent advice given to me by my good friend Veronica Harnish (author of "*Car Living When There Is No Other Choice*"): "So in that case, what I would do if I were a teen boy is to go to the local post office and buy postal money orders he can then address to/pay to himself and can later cash himself. It's easier and safer than keeping cash at home. Money orders never expire and can be bought for almost any amount for a usually less than $2 each. Every post office has money orders, so he doesn't have to go searching for retail locations like payday lender places, bank branches, or convenience stores. Also, if the money order is lost or stolen, and he has kept the receipt, it is replaceable. There's no age requirement to buy a money order. Money orders are small enough that they can be stored safely in a book or other place well-hidden. This lets the boy stay totally in control of his money without being 18 years old." (Thank you, Veronica. You rock, girl!)

When you are older, and you earn really good money, you can invest it in other than a savings account. First, however, before you invest that big money, be forewarned: The Government is going to want to you to pay taxes on your good income at least at the Federal level, and depending on where you live, on the State and Local levels as well. Failure to pay your taxes is the quickest way to get in trouble with the Government. The Internal Revenue Service (which handles tax payments for the Federal Government) is second only to the world's great militaries in terms of power. The IRS's power is virtually unlimited to come after you for your taxes. Don't fail to pay your taxes, or you will cause many problems in your life. There are software programs (like TurboTax) which can help you figure out your taxes owed. You can also try HR Block or Liberty Tax offices to help you. Sometimes local libraries have volunteers to help people such as you file their taxes. And who knows? You may get money *back* from the taxes you have already paid over the course of the year. Wouldn't that be excellent?!

You are never too young to start saving for your college education and retirement. Be sure of something when investing your hard-earned money: no one is ever going to care about your money as much as you do. Be careful about trusting professional money managers. They can make mistakes and steer you wrong and you lose your invested monies. Some may even be downright crooked and steal your money outright. Be careful with them! If you find yourself with extra money to invest, do your own research and find the best investments for you. A very famous and extremely rich investor, Warren Buffett, says that "you should never invest in something you don't understand". That is wise advice! Know where your hard-earned money is going in every investment you do.

Maybe you have no savings, and you need immediate cash. Do you have things you no longer want or need (like old CDs or DVDs)? Craigslist, LetGo, and eBay are great websites to sell items online in order to generate cash quickly. Going to a pawn shop is debatable, but since I have used them in the past to sell odd items, I don't protest against them. Do not use a pawn shop for a loan, however, as the fees are scandalous, and no loan is worth what the pawn shop will charge you for it. And, very important here, stay far, far away from Payday Loans and car-title (when you own a car) loan shops as well. They have outrageously humongous interest rates attached to the loans that they offer. A loan from one of these places snowballs until it gets so big that paying it back is almost impossible. (Personally, I think Payday and car titles lenders should be outlawed, as they especially prey on the poor people and broken families in our society. They are sharks!)

At a certain age you will be old enough to get a credit card. Be careful with credit cards. They can help you establish credit and come in handy for emergencies but use them only when necessary (like when ordering online). Always pay the balance off each month. If you can get 'points' for gift cards or cash-back from using a credit card or debit card, great, but don't let that motivate you to spend more (which is really what the credit card company or bank wants you to do). Instead of a credit card, use a debit card at your bank without an overdraft protection. Overdraft protection is like a credit card in that it is a high-interest loan from the bank if you charge more than what the balance is in your account. You don't need this. Getting into debt with credit cards or overdraft protection with your debit card is not good. It will be very difficult to ever pay this debt off. It's like a forest fire that generates its own weather system: your small monthly payments will never take care of the whole debt problem. Of course, those small monthly payments that you must make will inevitably get higher the more you owe. Pretty soon you find it hard to make those payments at all. So, watch out for credit cards and overdraft protection on debit cards. Note: If you do happen to get seriously in over your head in debt, search online for free debt counseling services that are available to you either over the phone or in your local area. There is no reason ever to pay a company to handle your debt servicing for you. Free debt counseling services are just as helpful.

Avoid debt by living below your means. This means being frugal. Being frugal is a state of mind that you can develop now while you are young with little money. There are many books, videos, and blogs on living frugally. You don't need to buy the books - go to your library and borrow them. This actually is rule #1 in living frugally: get to know your local library system well – something that is really advantageous to living in North America. Once you establish the habit of being frugal, it will serve you well all your life. One way to start with being frugal is always buy for quality. As my favorite uncle, a farmer (now deceased – may he rest in peace), once told me, "I am too poor to buy cheap tools and machinery". What he meant is, if he had bought cheap equipment, it would break and become useless so many times that the costs of fixing or replacing it would be greater than if he had decided in the first place to buy quality equipment. He bought quality and it saved him money over the long-term. Unlike many farmers during the 1980s, my uncle survived and thrived and did not lose his farm. A wise man with money, he was.

When deciding whether to spend your money or save it, make sure you can distinguish between a 'want' and a 'need'. Soap and shampoo to keep yourself clean, and notebooks for school are needs. A Sony PlayStation, a skateboard, or a Coca-Cola are wants. Make 'wise buying decisions' an important skill to learn. You will manage your spending better than 90% of North Americans if you can stop and ask yourself right before you purchase something, *"Do I really need this? Or is it just a passing want? How have I lived my life until now without it?"* I can guarantee you, little brother, that if you don't buy what is in front of you and wait three days before purchasing this 'want', you will end up saying to yourself that it really wasn't something necessary for your life. Saving the money will be more valuable and interesting for you. That doesn't mean you should never buy 'wants' (like a Sony PlayStation or skateboard, they are pretty cool) to enjoy. Knowing that many 'wants' (like a bag of potato chips from 7-11 or a McDonald's Big Mac) are fleeting and temporary will 'keep money from burning a hole in your pocket' (help you to save money and not to spend it).

An unfortunate and big problem you will have to deal with all your life is that advertisers are fighting very hard to make you spend money. Advertising is everywhere, as you surely know by now. It cannot be avoided in modern society. Learn now, though, to avoid being sucked in by advertising that offers the 'biggest', the 'best', or the 'newest' of anything. Those items will always without a doubt be the costliest to you. It takes a lot of diligence to master avoiding the control of advertising over you, but you can do it if you are serious about managing your money well.

The 'newest' does not need to be the 'best' in your life. Shop at thrift stores like Goodwill or The Salvation Army (or other types of thrift stores in your area) for permanent things you need like furniture, clothes and shoes, and such things as new notebooks or pens. Shopping at thrift stores is a great idea in our society for three reasons: 1. They benefit local charities, 2. You save money (oftentimes lots of money off the price of an equivalent new item, with little difference in the item you can buy and its newer, latest version), 3. You cut down on world consumption by 'recycling' used items. Have a good eye for what you buy at thrift stores, however, because something this already used may have poor quality. This is normally not the case at the larger, well-known thrift stores, but it can happen that you get a bad or low-quality product at a thrift store. Thrift stores are fun to shop in because they can be like a treasure hunt to find what you need at a really good price. My wife buys my children's clothing at the local Goodwill thrift store (and until you have your own children, you have no idea the high cost to clothe a kid from infanthood up to teenage years). You can't tell the difference in the quality of the items she hunts and shops for from anything which can be bought at the expensive stores Macy's and Nordstrom at the local expensive mall. (Well, at least I can't tell any difference.) On thing though: don't buy sneakers at thrift stores if you plan to do any physical activity in them because used sneakers are worn-out and no longer have the protection your feet need. If you want them for 'the look' to walk around in, then it is okay to buy used.

Buying new sneakers or any clothing for 'the look' is a waste of money. Did you know that most name brand sneakers are made in the same one factory in China? No matter what name brand or what price of sneakers you buy, they are almost always going to be of the same quality. Only the styles will be different. If you wait 'a season' for the certain latest style of something (sneakers, electronics, clothes, etc.) to pass, the next year that same product will have a very substantial price reduction as the store is eager to get rid of it quickly. In all cases, use the internet to research the different prices and varieties of anything you want to buy, new or used. eBay and Craigslist are great places to buy items if you know specifically what you are looking for. As always, 'buyer beware' of scams or quality issues.

Some things you just have to buy new, if only for sanitary reasons. If you have to buy new clothing (such as underwear, swimsuits, hats and socks), offbeat discount stores like Ross, Marshalls, and TJ Maxx are the best bet for your money. Outlet brand-name stores can sometimes be a bargain if you know what you are looking for specifically and have shopped around already in other places. However, brand-name outlets are so universal now that they often sell a lot of damaged and low-quality items for barely less than a new item at their regular store.

Dollar Stores are a great place for necessities such as soap, shampoo, and temporary-use odds and ends (be wary of quality). Pharmacy stores can sometimes be inexpensive as well. Check and see if the store you want to buy in has an app for discounts. If you are going to be buying food, avoid the convenience stores like 7-11, Wawa, or Circle-K. The price-mark-ups on items in these stores are huge and not worth the 'convenience'. It is better to shop at a big-name grocery store, or big box store like Walmart or Target, especially if you have a manufacturer's or store coupon. Generic and store brand items for food, paper products, toiletries, and over-the-counter medicines cost much less than a special brand name product. Did you know that generic items are usually made and packaged in the exact same factory as the brand name item? It's true!

Using your local or school library was mentioned above. There you can get books, DVDs, CDs, and audiobooks for free to borrow, but make sure you return them by the due dates or you will have to pay a fine. Your favorite magazines are also available to read at many libraries, so no need to pay money to subscribe to them. Many libraries will let you use their computers for a set period of time each day for free to surf or do research on the internet. If you have internet at home, there is no need for you to go out and buy the latest CD or pay to download the latest songs and movies. Youtube.com will show you music videos of the latest songs by your favorite artists for in return only watching a few seconds of advertising (which you know by now should be 'turned off' in your mind, anyway).

Of course, if you do want something bad enough, save up for it. If you don't have the money right now for it and for whatever reason you have to have it right now, borrow the money from someone close to you. Make sure you pay them back fully to retain their trust. Under no circumstances should you ever steal (shoplift) the item you want. Shoplifting is a quick way to get yourself into juvenile detention (jail for teens) and deeply into other problems with the law. Stealing is not just against the law. It is breaking one of the Ten Commandments given to us by God.

There is still more you can do with your money than saving and buying. One of the best things you can do with some of your money is to donate to charities regularly. Giving a small part of your income regularly to a charity will help you feel better about yourself. You will be helping people in need, and, believe it or not, God will reward you in some way in return. Some churches ask that you donate 10% of your income (called 'tithing') to them, but this depends on the church you go to, and is certainly not a hard-fast rule you have to hold yourself accountable to. I do not recommend giving money to panhandlers (people begging on street corners or at street intersections) as often they will spend the money on alcohol, drugs, or cigarettes. Give instead to charities which help these people, such as a local homeless shelter or soup kitchen. You can also do what my children and I do. We buy cookies at McDonald's (three for a dollar plus tax) or small bottles of water and give them to people panhandling. We even buy McDonald's cookies for the local police officers and the military personnel whom we see in the restaurant near us. My children learn what charity and giving of yourself freely are all about, and they also learn to respect people in uniform.

A final word: understand that money is a 'divider'. That is, money can make or break your relationships with other people, depending on how you view it in your own life. People sometimes do awful things to get money. Money can make you, too, do things you don't really want to do. Respect money, and it will return respect to you. That's a valuable lesson right there that makes reading this book worthwhile.

Chapter IX – Other Boys

You have a basic need deep inside of you. That need, even if you don't realize it well, is to belong and be respected. There is nothing wrong with having that need. To want to belong to a group of other boys is a wonderful thing. I am 100% sure that not having it fulfilled completely will make you feel empty and insecure. But where can you get this need filled correctly? Let's look first at a wrong way. Right now, I am sure there is a local gang near where you live trying to recruit you to join them. That desire to join them is the element of wanting to belong to something meaningful. Gangs survive and thrive on this need which boys like you have. However, you this is a bad idea. Rather than the corner gang, better for you to find a group that is well suited to help guide you to become a good, Godly man. In some other cultures in the world, there are 'bands' or 'tribes' that raise boys to become men. Unfortunately, we don't have these kinds of tribes in society in North America. Many grown men would say that we as a society and you as an individual probably would be better off if we did. The group(s) that you join today, and how you behave to other boys in that group, will set your destiny and manhood in motion like a freight-train busting down the tracks with unstoppable power. That is what this chapter will mainly discuss and focus on: how to build your good character and personality through the company of boys and men you are with.

"I'd rather face an army of lions led by a sheep, than an army of sheep led by a lion."

Alexander the Great (world conqueror)

Men were made to be leaders, protectors, and providers. That is what God intended. You can be a leader someday, too. You can be a leader in business, politics, education, or sports (just to name a few examples where good leaders are needed in this world). You can also be the leader of your family someday as a husband to your wife and father to your children. How you become a good leader begins with where you set your time and efforts today with regards to other good boys and men.

A few questions to think about:

What kind of boys do you hang around with in your free time? Who are your main homeboys these days? What kind of older men do you look up to as being positive forces in the world? Who is the man (or men) you see in life whom you want to be like when you grow up? Are there any patterns to the answers to these questions that you can recognize? I hope so.

These are the questions you should be asking yourself as your go through life hanging with your best buddies and making decisions on what kind of man you want to be when you are older. Now, today, is the time to focus on these questions. Not tomorrow or next week – it's too late then. Sooner or later the boys you hang out with now, today, will affect your character in some way, either for good or for bad. The men you look up to today are going to influence your behaviors and values in life as well. Let me ask you a quick question: If you have a clean basket full of juicy red apples, and one apple at the bottom is rotten, what happens at the end of one week? Do you think the good, juicy apples make the rotten one 'good'? Or do you understand well that the rotten apple will in turn make all the other 'good' apples rotten? That is what happens every time, my friend. The same goes for you with regards to all the boys you associate with. If you hang on the corner with the boys who shoplift, sell drugs, carry weapons, impregnate girls, etc., then, my friend, soon enough you, too, will be doing the same horrible actions. It's unavoidable. You cannot help yourself from being corrupted by such bad boys. And that's a bad thing. Instead, if you find some good boys at the local Boys & Girls Club, or on a local sports team you can join to play with, or (even better) at a good church with a teenage ministry to be a part, then you will have their good influence 'rub off' on you and keep you on the narrow path of goodness and holiness. This, too, is unavoidable. And that's a good thing.

Groups are made of friends. Friends are individuals first, then part of the group. It is good to have one really good friend to influence you whom you can trust. He can be your best friend. Here is a quick list of some sample questions to think about with regards to how you interact with your best friend:

Do you respect your best friend's girlfriend as HIS girlfriend, or do you flirt with her?

Do you build up your best friend with encouragement, or do you tear him down with insults?

Do you help him clean up if he invites you over to his house for lunch, or do you leave without saying 'thank you' and lending a hand?

Do you butt into his private conversations he may be having with his girlfriend or someone else?

Do you pay your fair share, and possibly even part of his, if you go out for milkshakes and french-fries at the diner?

Do you show up late when he invites you somewhere, or are you on time, if not early, to meet him at the place he asked you to join him?

As you can guess, what you do for your friend and how you treat him reflects what kind of person you really are. How you choose to speak to him is of the utmost importance. You need to be honest with him, be sincere with him, show yourself to have integrity with your words, and treat him as an individual different from you. If you are not honest with him (or anyone) and tell him lies, then you will not establish trust. Trust is key for continued cooperation on any activities you would like his help on. If you are not sincere with him, and you act towards him in a different way than you actually are, think, or feel, then this is like lying to him as well. If you have integrity with your friend, then your actions will be positive, and you will do what you said you would do for him. He will then in turn do well for you. Probably the most important aspect to learn about friendship: you have to like your friend just for who he is and nothing more. He isn't going to change for you, no matter how hard you try to change him. There is an old saying: An enemy can be your friend if you will let him be who he is.

We read about it an above paragraph. There are bad boys – rotten apples - out there, everywhere in the wide world, just waiting to cause trouble and mayhem. There are boys who will do bad things to you and those around you whom you love. This hasn't changed since the Fall of Man. Evil exists in the world, and nothing in the world is capable of putting an end to Evil until the Lord comes again.

This dude I know dissed me (or bullied me) bad! And now I want to get back at him!

I know, I know. You gotta get 'respect', gotta show you are a tough, hard guy, all because you were dissed. No normal rational behavior here, no basic human values or morals, just a self-imposed 'chip on the shoulder' and constant need to prove you are a hard, bad ass. This is just more of the misguided 'street code'. Sorry, little brother, but that 'street code' is wrong thinking plain and simple. If you get back at the one who hurt you, you are nothing more than a street punk who injured another human. (I don't mean he didn't hurt your ego first, but he didn't damage you physically, at least not permanently). And I will go so far to tell you that if you take revenge, you will be known as an uneducated loser like him (remember the chapter on doing stupid things?). Hurting someone who hurt you starts a bad cycle that may not end. The Japanese have a saying: If you want to take revenge, start by digging two graves.

But that doesn't mean I am telling you not to defend yourself from another boy is physically hurting you. Not in the slightest. You have every right – and the law is on your side – to defend yourself when attacked. Dealing with difficult boys (bullies) in your life can be handled by taking up a martial arts class or doing some weight-lifting to bulk up. The best way to 'street-fight' is by knowing how to wrestle, because inevitably all street-fights end up happening off your feet on the ground. You can also run away if attacked. One old saying goes, "He who doesn't fight and runs away, lives to fight another day." Other boys may call you chicken but running away may prevent you from being jumped by multiple attackers such as a gang. In that instance, you are guaranteed to lose if you try to fight them all. There is no shame in running away from a fight. Believe me. None at all.

You are allowed to get as angry as you want your feelings to feel when you are dissed. You can be outrageously furious even, if you think you need to feel that way. But you do not have the right to hurt anyone else, emotionally or physically, because of your anger. Learning to diffuse your anger is a rite of passage all teen boys must pass before entering into adulthood. Mature people deal with their anger in positive ways. So, you are angry. Go ride a bicycle up hill or go run around the block five times. You can do almost anything physical, except throw or break things, to diffuse the bad feelings you have now against the dude who dissed you.

A relationship without disagreements is only found between a shepherd and his sheep. Why do I make this silly claim? Because with you and other boys there can be no intimacy without conflict. That is just how relations among human beings' work. Resolve your disagreements with others as soon as you can as time does not 'heal all wounds'. When issues are not resolved, anger and bitterness take root in the heart, and cleaning that garbage out takes more time and emotional work than dealing with the issues in the first place. Decide to 'agree to disagree' and compromise if necessity compels you to. Sometimes you and a friend will come to a stalemate where both of you think you are 'right' with no compromise possible. You are best served then to take a step back and refrain from any further confrontation. You in your humility are thus the 'greater man'. In this manner, the relationship can be rebuilt, and it naturally follows that you will be the leader in the rebuilding. What have you lost then? Absolutely nothing.

Whether you mean to or not, you are sometimes going to hurt your friends on occasion with your words or your actions. If you do wrong to your homie or anyone else (like your mother), be quick to apologize humbly and ask sincerely for their forgiveness. You don't want to lose the trust of those boys who are important to you, because a good friend can be there for your entire life. I have two good friends I have had going on 27 years now, and I wouldn't trade the friendships I have with them for anything. Sometimes I need to apologize to them even though we have known each other for so long because I hurt them either accidentally or in a fit of frustration when I lash out. Lashing out is wrong in itself, of course, but starting with a sincere apology afterwards repairs the relationship. Apologize, or the relationship is forever damaged. This is just common sense, but you would be surprised at the number of teen boys, and even adult men, who fail to ask for forgiveness of others close to them. These men are wrong as they just strut along in their life with pride in their hearts, thus losing a valued friend. It happens time and time again, unfortunately, in this cold world we live in. It is preventable if you are humble enough and care enough about the other boy to show them you do care.

Remember: the best way to get a friend is to be one.

Chapter X - Girls and Women

Boys and men want to be respected. Girls and women want to be loved. That is a big, defining difference between the sexes. And it has been that way since the first men and women were placed on the earth by our God.

To understand women when you are older, you may want to read a book titled "*Men are from Mars, Women are from Venus*" by John Gray. It has its critics, but it is well worth taking the time to read to get perspective on the relationship situation between a man and a woman. Men and women, boys and girls, have different ways of thinking and viewing the world, and that is okay. There is nothing wrong with this. God made us in His Image, and both men and women have characteristics of God that the opposite sex does not have. In this complex world we live in, it is beneficial to have two different minds working together in marriage to solve the problems of survival, raising children, and planning a future together. I know my life would not be functionally the same and definitely would be sadly incomplete, if I didn't share it with the greatest love of my life: my wife of seventeen (and hopefully many more) years, Julia.

Therefore, respect the other gender as it takes two of us to make this world work out right. Girls are different from boys, and women are different from men. Understand that now. We think differently, we act differently, and we are built physically differently (this last part I probably didn't even need to tell you). No one can change what nature orders. Sometimes women might appear or want to think like men do, but they won't stay that way. They aren't necessarily wrong in their thinking and acting, just different from your own thoughts and actions. It is really stupid to expect a girl to think and act like a boy, and vice-versa. Movies love to tell those stories, but they are all entirely pure fiction. You have to work it out in your relationships with women. That can start well by compromise inspired by love, and not by simple retreat or surrender.

Girls and women of any age love attention. Your mother in particular is someone who should get a lot of your attention and praise in life. She may be trying to do for you what she was not meant to do: trying to raise you to become a man. But, here's the thing, she can't. A woman cannot raise her son to be a man, no matter how hard or well she tries. You need to be around other men to learn to be a man. Your mother may be good, even Godly. She most likely is doing all she can to provide for you (just as my own mother raised four children under the age of 12 all on her own), so she needs your support and cooperation in all things. Don't fight or argue unnecessarily with her. Don't disrespect her. At the very least she gave you life. If she is there for you as best as she can be, in return you owe her respect. That is what God requires in one of His Commandments to us: that we respect our parents, no matter what bad things they have done to us. Yes, your mother is going to make you angry and frustrated sometimes, especially when she 'doesn't get where you're coming from' as a teenage boy. But I guarantee she is doing her best to help you and support you. Don't push her away. Accept her as part of your life. She may be hurting at the loss of her husband/partner (your father), so anything you can do to relieve her of that pain would be invaluable. God then will surely reward you for it. Be mature and treat your mother well. She will notice your good interactions with her as a sign of your maturity, and you two will build a strong bond that will last an entire lifetime. And believe me, that strong bond you can have with your mother is worth more than gold. I know this all too well, as I had to rely on my own mother (may she rest in peace) to help me much in my teen years.

In all ways financially look out for your mother as well. Since the 1960s, women have started to get better employment opportunities (and that is, no doubt, a very good thing), but one of the negative consequences of this is that the majority of children in the USA now no longer have the income of a married father to rely on. Probably your mother's money alone is being used to support you and your siblings. If she gives you some of her money to you for your own wants and desires, use it wisely and make her proud.

There are several other ways to respect your mother. Here are some: 1. learn to say you are sorry to your mother, no matter how hard it is to say it; 2. don't go to bed angry at your mother; 3. kiss your mother every day and tell her you love her, even if at that moment you don't feel like it; 3. be happy and laugh with your mother even if you are not in the mood or it seems idiotic at that moment to do so; 4. never take your mother for granted, as God can take her away from you at any time. The short time you have with your mother on this planet is precious. Learn to use it productively, as a good, real son does, and you will make everyone in your family happy and joyful and Godly.

One thing needs to be carefully considered here with regards to your mother. As I described above, your mother is most likely 'wounded' at the absence of your father. This wound is primarily emotional. Because it is her nature as a woman, she will seek any way possible to heal this wound. That may involve you in a bad way. One problematic situation that can happen between a teen boy and his single mother is that he becomes her 'savior' or her 'boyfriend'. It goes without saying that this kind of flaw in the relationship between a mother and her teen son can cause all kinds of problems for both of you. If you suspect you are in such a flawed relationship with your mother, especially if you feel guilty in that you must 'save' her somehow, you are going to need some counseling, preferably from a trusted man such as a member of the church clergy. You must understand that in no way are you responsible for your mother or her situation. In the same way, you must not 'be there for her' as a husband or other adult male figure can and should have. You are far too young and vulnerable right now to let this kind of flawed situation happen to you. I will repeat it: if you feel guilty in any way for your mother's situation, whether she places that burden on you intentionally or not, seek guidance from a trusted adult man. I cannot stress the importance of this enough! Both you and your mother will suffer greatly if the problem is not addressed and dealt with appropriately. That is something I will tell you is 100% guaranteed, my little friend, because I lived it myself.

Respect each older woman you know or meet as if she were your own mother or grandmother. This includes aunts, teachers, schools' principals, police officers, and any other older women you may come across. The woman you respect today may be the one who helps you reach your goals tomorrow. Women can be very helpful to young men such as yourself if you show them the proper respect they are due. If you don't respect them, then you can be sure you will get zero help from them. Women are different from men in that they have very long memories and will hold it against you that you disrespected them. Do the right thing. Respect the older women in your life.

For dealing with girls your age now, life can be tricky. Better to put off dating as long as you can and focus on other areas of growing up. There will be plenty of time later for dating. You can date a lot of girls in your time before marriage. When you do date, treat each girl you date as the 'special one for you', and always, always, always date them one at a time. Having multiple girlfriends is a good way to ruin your reputation and blow out any trust that girls and women may have for you. Respect each girl you date as if she were your sister. How do you want your sister to be treated by her boyfriend? Do the same. Kiss your girlfriend only when you are ready to ask her to marry you (again, this is still many years from now).

Other boys around you are bragging about how many girls they have fooled around with or even slept with. You can rest assured that this bragging is most likely bull-crap. (And that is the only time I will use that word in this book). Simple-minded men like to brag about their sexual conquests, real or imagined. Real or lies, it is disrespectful to females to talk in this manner. As for you, don't ever allow yourself to be 'stuck' in a compromising position with a girl, such as together alone in your bedroom or hers. You both will be fighting your powerful hormones and sexual lusts. Inevitably you both will lose that fight. Sex outside of marriage brings unwanted pregnancies, diseases transmitted between partners, and broken hearts.

Marriage is a very long way off for you. The longer you put it off, the better. You shouldn't even think about it until you are financially stable and at least in your 20s. It is worth noting here a few things about marriage. *The following is just 'food for thought' that you can think about for the next several years before you are married.* After you become married, there are some basic and not so basic rules to pay attention to. The first and foremost is, of course, 'forsaking all other women'. Yes, when you are married, you are done with dating and being involved emotionally or physically with all other women. There is then one and only one woman in your life: your wife. She even takes precedence over your own mother in your decision making and life's issues. That is the way God intended it. Breaking the God-given rule of 'one man-one woman' will only lead to disaster for you, your wife, your marriage, and if you have them, your children. Very little can be done to recover yourself once you break this rule, as the consequences are usually irreversible. Women, as lovely in heart as they are, can be very forgiving, but that doesn't mean they must be forgiving. Learn from other weasel-men before you who ruined their own lives by cheating on their wives. These were not 'real men' by any means. They were still young boys who, like Peter Pan, never grew up and only sought pleasure, not serious honest commitment. The damage they have caused in society is probably partly to blame for your own current situation. Fatherless children often come from callous, worthless men.

One of the best pleasures in life for a man is to have a relationship with a woman. You can be married to a woman someday, have one as your mother, or be a good friend to one at school now. Like all relationships, your character shows with how you treat women. Show the best person you can be by loving and respecting all women in your life. All women will praise you when you do.

Chapter XI – Your Body

A clean mind and a healthy body work well together. As we will see in the next chapter, your mind is critical to your well-being. In this chapter, we are going to look at your body and how to keep yourself physically well.

Your physical body is going through some major changes as you read this book. I won't go into details here, first because you already know and see some of those changes happening to you. Second, there is a good book I recommend you get at the library: *"What's Happening to Me?"*, by Peter Mayle. This book will answer your questions about puberty and the changes you see happening to you during your early teenage years. If your library doesn't have it on the shelves, ask the librarian to get a copy for you.

The Greeks had it right: a good body tends to mean a good brain and spirit. Some arrogant jocks might be like "Oh, whatever, sporto!". Still, men are indeed happy when they exert themselves physically. When a man exercises, endorphins are released in the body into the bloodstream. These are natural attitude adjusters which will make you feel good. They also make you think better and clearer. Yeah, most jocks are pretty smart after all just for exercising their hearts out. Therefore, I say, exercise! It is usually either hard to get started or hard to keep going. By doing something physical for a couple of weeks or so, you will quickly establish it as a habit. It will become a natural part of your regular life routine. Once you form that good habit of going to the gym or playing basketball at the playground, when you miss it, you really miss it.

Eat good food. Avoid junk. Add fruits, vegetables, some breads and cereals, and some fish or lean meat to your daily meals. Stay away from sugar and greasy foods. It really is the only way to be a healthy eater. Living requires you to drink lots of water. Exercise requires even more water. Whether or not to drink a chocolate milkshake or a Diet Coca-Cola with lunch today isn't going to make much of a difference... unless you are a diabetic. Why do I tell you this example? Because choices and decisions about health (as well as many other areas of life) are different and individualized for each and every person. Your choices about eating and drinking foods which affect your health are yours alone. You own them. No one can make your healthy decisions for you.

Go see a doctor and a dentist, once per year if you can. If you have no insurance and your family cannot afford it, ask at your school's guidance counselor's office about finding a medical clinic where you can get a physical exam at low or no cost. Befriend your doctor. He or she wants what is best for you. When your doctor gives you any advice or medication to take, do it faithfully. A doctor in the United States goes through many tough years of schooling and training just to help you. Listen to them as you would listen to your own mother's good advice. It is also good to ask questions to your doctor. There is a famous television commercial where a man is at a local electronics store, and he asks multiple questions about the cell phone he is about to buy. Cut to the scene where he is in his doctor's office, and the doctor asks him if he has any questions. He gives a soft answer, "No." This is a sad waste of a resource men can benefit from. Doctors are a wealth of information about our bodies and minds that we can tap into. If we let that learning opportunity pass us by, we are doing a big disservice to ourselves. So, take the time to make a list of questions you want to know about your health and your body before you see a doctor. Not only will he or she be impressed, but the doctor will take all the extra time necessary to help you in your search to find out more about yourself. Under no circumstances should you risk your health, even if you think the medical problem you have is small or you lack the funds to cover the medical bills. You might 'feel' okay, even when your doctor tells you otherwise. Many times, small health problems can become worse very quickly, and that may require more medical help than originally needed. This results in a possible emergency room visit or hospitalization, and most definitely bigger health care bills. Better to get the right treatment as soon as possible. If there are big medical bills (because there was no free-clinic available to you), negotiate with the health care provider's billing office to reduce them and pay them over time.

Adequate and proper sleep habits as a teenager are crucial to good physical health and a stable mind. If you stay up all night playing video games highly caffeinated on Red Bull and then go to school the next day, this is not just unhealthy (especially for your heart and brain) but for sure you are going to fall asleep at your desk in class. As a young teenager especially, you need lots of sleep as your body goes through puberty. Lack of sleep will lead your body to being more susceptible to colds and the flu. Just as you need structure during your day (eating breakfast every morning, going to school at the same time daily, soccer practice in the afternoons, etc.), you need a regular sleep routine that you do not deviate from. Don't oversleep on weekends or say you will 'catch up' on sleep you missed during the week on the weekends. That doesn't work in the human body. Better to establish an early bedtime daily and get up after a good night's sleep ready to start your day well and bright. If you are tired during the day, then it is okay to take a brief nap. But don't make taking naps a habit, or you will find it very difficult to break it. You might be tempted to sleep too much. To stop this temptation, get up and take a cold shower, or go outside if it is winter in shorts and a t-shirt until the temptation leaves you. The temptation to 'love sleep' can be very powerful. You don't want it to control you.

People have the 'breath of life' in their nostrils. Learn how to breathe deep from your diaphragm, in through your nose and out through your mouth. Good breathing techniques will help you play sports and do other physical activities better. Good breathing also overcomes anxiety and sadness and calms many overheated situations you may have with other people. Breathing deeply relaxes you during stressful situations. Breathe in on a count of four. Hold your breath for a count of four. Then exhale on a count of four. Imagine the stress leaving you as you breathe deep and exhale.

Drugs and substances. Some are illegal in our society, and some cause a habitual abuse of valid doctors' prescriptions. It makes no difference here. When you make your body and mind feel good ("escapism", for a very brief moment, until you crash) from drugs, you are damaging your body, mind and spirit at the same time. Abuse of drugs is permanently damaging in these areas of the self. Drugs can also lead to death through accidental overdose. As of my writing this now, legal marijuana use 'recreationally' or by doctor's prescription is advancing in our society. Also, at the time of this writing, a report from the University of California-Davis came out that said that long-term smoking of marijuana makes a person (and I am using the directly quoted words here from the study) *"more likely to become a loser"*. The same is true not just for legal or illegal marijuana, but also for other illegal drugs, such as heroin, methamphetamine, cocaine, flakka, ecstasy, and bath salts (to name a few of the popular ones today). Prescription drugs, when abused, are detrimental to your well-being. What negatives can happen to you, little brother, if you decide to indulge yourself in drug abuse? You will certainly experience downward social mobility (meaning your friends will tend to be losers, too), serious financial problems, bad medical issues, and potential problems with the law and homelessness. Do yourself a favor: stay far away from drugs. There is nothing, I repeat, nothing, to be gained from partaking in substance abuse.

Alcohol, though legal for people over the age 21 (no, you are not there yet, not even close), is also a drug. When you are old enough for alcohol, drink only in moderation. Abuse of alcohol can lead to serious damage to the body, mind, social situations, and lead to the other negatives listed above for drug abuse. If you have knowledge of alcoholism in your family (your mother, an aunt/uncle, or perhaps you know about your father's alcoholism), then it is highly likely you, too, will suffer from alcoholism. Maybe your family has a history of alcoholism, and you think for one minute that you can control your own drinking of alcohol through sheer willpower. I will tell you, little brother, that you are dead wrong. For an alcoholic, one drink, even 'socially', is too much and too little at the same time. Don't risk ruining your life. It is best to stay away from alcohol, even if you aren't susceptible to alcoholism. By the way, if your friends are drinking at a young age, and they are pushing you to join them, as Nancy Reagan (wife to President Ronald Reagan) preached in the 1980s, "Just say no". To drink when you are underage, and your brain has not fully developed yet is just plain stupid.

Do you understand now that "escapism" through drugs or alcohol will lead to all kinds of problems? Believe it. You may even see it in your own world. Take the advice from someone who in his youth 'played with fire' and has seen in other people the serious problems substance and alcohol abuse can cause.

Now I will touch on a very sensitive issue about your body and your respect for it: *masturbation*. Simply: don't do it. Not once even. There is no quicker way to destroy your relationships with your friends, other men, and even girls and women, than by masturbating. It is sin, plain and simple, and you reap what you sow in this world (you may have heard someone say that very phrase to you before). Once you start masturbating, for even only a few times, the temptation to do it more will grow like weeds in your heart. The longer this goes on, the harder it will be to stop doing it and pull out the weeds. And believe me, my little brother, when you make it a habit, you will desperately want to stop it because you will feel and know its destruction in you. But it will be too late - you not be able to stop it on your own without counseling and prayer from others. The best thing you can do when you are tempted to masturbate is to get up and take a cold shower, or if it is winter go out into the cold in shorts and a t-shirt, until the hot temptation passes. It is a good idea to talk about this temptation with your mentor or a member of the clergy. You probably should not discuss it with your friends, unless they are of the same belief that is a very sinful habit. It also helps to know what negatives mood or feelings you have when you are tempted. This will go a long way in the prevention of the temptation even coming. That is just how your body and mind work together in this. As said above, talking about it with a trusted mentor will be very helpful. Be honest about it with him as you discuss it. No need to be embarrassed or ashamed or feel guilty talking about it because every man has this to deal with. Preventing it from happening in the first place is the best way to go. If you do happen to do it, be sure to confess that you did it to a trusted mentor or a friend who, again, is of the same belief that is it is a grave sin.

God has given you only one body in this world. Be good to your body. It will last you a lifetime if you take good care of it!

Chapter XII – Your Mind

As the television publicity said in the 1970s, "A mind is a terrible thing to waste". Reading materials, watching a screen, and listening to music are some mind inputs that can affect your life for good or for bad depending on what you choose. There is a word computer programmer's use: GIGO. It means "garbage in-garbage out". This means that if the computer program is garbage, the end result will not be what was intended by the programmer. The same is true with your own mind. What you put into your mind determines what comes out of it. For example: if you choose to watch pornography on the internet, you are going to develop an addiction to it and possibly an addiction to masturbation as well. Both addictions are destructive to your mind, body and soul. If you listen to hateful rap music that promotes anti-cop, anti-women themes, then you, too, are going to become a hateful young man. If you play violent video games all day long, there is a good chance you will end up a very violent young man.

Your mind is not like a sieve that filters the good from the bad. It is more like a melting-pot container. Whatever you put into it, you can never take out, and it blends everything together into one mix of thoughts. Bad experiences and choices will always come into play here. If you do the GIGO thing, then expect that you are going to become a criminal someday, and end up in prison, or worse, dead. If you don't believe any of this, talk with your mentor if he knows any stories of boys who self-destructed at a young age thus ruining their own and many others' lives, all because of the choices they made in the materials they put into their minds. Examples of boys self-destructing from what they put into their minds are shown each and every day in the news. The prisons are full of grown men who started exactly where you are right now: they made the wrong decisions as boys as to what to fill their minds with. Now they are 'paying back' for those bad choices. (See Jeremy Sly's quote at the beginning of the book.) Don't let this happen to you!

Time and again it has been shown through various psychological studies that what goes into a boy's brain determines a large part of who he is to be and become. Listen to the different modern music radio stations, and you will hear the garbage society is peddling. Some music is for the vain glory of the singers and their creators. Usually this kind of music is destructive to the soul. The kind of music you listen to should be helpful to calm your mind and body. It will help you to focus when you are studying, and it will also keep your mind from being filled with much of the garbage and destruction society is trying to sell to you. So, it is up to you to make the right choices as to what you will put into your brain. Non-hateful, non-violent, and non-vulgar music is beneficial. Jazz, Christian-themed, and classical music are some examples of what you should be listening to. You may not have a strong taste for such good music now, but you can develop a liking over time.

Reading wholesome literature is good for you. There are hundreds of good books, both contemporary and classic, that you can read and learn about life from. Sagas of people's lives and the difficulties they overcame will be especially beneficial for you to read to learn about who you are and what you can become. Both good music and good literature will build your mind and help it to create beauty in the world rather than be fatefully attracted to all the evils around you. Mark Twain (a good writer himself) said that "A man who can read good books and doesn't has no advantage over the man who cannot read". Millionaires and billionaires all agree that constantly reading good materials helped them along the way to becoming wealthy. So, take the time - start today - to read something educational and beneficial to your life. This book you have in your hands is a good start. A book on investing and creating wealth, or on finding a job, or on creating your own business, can do wonders for you for your entire life. Once you build the habit of reading good books, you will indeed find it more interesting than playing violent video games or listening to bad music.

As far as screen time goes, this is probably the most powerful media influence in our society. In my opinion, television shows are all useless trash and a waste of time. There is nothing shown on television which can build you up. (Okay, maybe sports are okay to watch. But not all sports. There is nothing beneficial about watching WrestleMania or UFC.) All R-rated movies and many PG-13 movies should be off your list of what to watch. Documentary video DVD's from the library to learn from are beneficial for you like good books.

The internet is a tool which is full of information that can be readily accessible in seconds to help you with your homework, research, or find something interesting to learn about. There are over a billion pages on the internet you can learn good things from, all because you can read English. The internet is also full of trash and evil. You know what I am talking about here. Those websites showing pornography or violent videos are of no benefit to you, not at all. Pornography is a severe problem in North America and around the world, and many men are hooked to it out of their own control (see the section in <u>Chapter XI – Your Body</u> on masturbation to understand this better). At all costs, do everything you can to avoid getting sucked into the pornography trap. Don't even 'dabble' in it. Once you fall into porn's grasp, it is all but impossible to get out of it without outside professional help. Even then for some men it's impossible to heal from it. Choose wisely what you look at on the screen. The same can be said about the damage from pornographic magazines. Yes, *The Sports Illustrated Swimsuit Issue* should also be avoided as it is too explicit.

This is where your mind is built at its very core: every image (and sound) you put in your mind can never be erased. No matter how faint it may become it will always be there. The choices you make today as to what to look at on a screen or page will have far-reaching effects on all areas of your life. This also means that you should not entertain sexual fantasies rolling around in your mind. Those, too, can lead to destruction through bad behaviors. Let's be clear about this: your actions will for sure follow what you put into your mind and what you spend your time thinking about. Be wise and choose carefully.

Your mental health needs to be nourished and cared for just like your physical health. Go ahead and feel all your emotions, not just the good ones. Really, really feel them, even if they suck to feel. There will be feelings you have that are painful, but you must feel them, or they will bottle up and not come out. I cannot stress the importance of this enough (based on my own sorry experiences). If you bottle up your emotions deep inside of you, you may eventually explode and that will result in other problems arising. Not dealing with your emotions will develop serious mental health problems which can possibly continue throughout your entire life. Psychiatrists (doctors who deal with mental health) all agree that many of the adults who have mental health problems are this way due to having suffered through serious childhood trauma and abuse. These people never processed the negative feelings that resulted. If you don't deal with how you need to feel now for any bad situations you are going through, then for sure you are setting yourself up for personal emotional disaster later in life. One thing to remember, however: you can feel any way you want or need to, any emotion is okay to feel, but you cannot hurt anyone else (physically or emotionally) with your hurt feelings and emotions. As is often said, "Hurt people, hurt people." Don't let this happen in your life. Other people should not have to suffer just because you're having a bad day. Deal with your bad emotions in a constructive, healthy way. Strenuous physical activity is a great way to blow off anger, sadness, and frustrations. Go for a run around the block or ride your bicycle uphill. In contrast, eating a box of Oreo cookies is not a good way to deal with bad emotions.

We all get sad sometimes. We get 'the blues' after our girlfriend breaks up with us or when we get a bad grade on the biology exam we studied so hard for. These briefs bouts of negativity are unavoidable for everyone. But, if you find yourself really down and sad for a period longer than, say, two weeks, you may be suffering from clinical depression. Having depression is one of the most grossly misunderstood medical issues in our society today. People – your friends and family - will tell you to 'snap out of it' or 'shake it off', when you know quite well that isn't going to happen. These people may mean well, but they are not mental health professionals, and they cannot help you now. If you suspect you have clinical depression, you are definitely going to need outside professional help. You cannot overcome it on your own. Most importantly, medicating yourself with drugs or alcohol is only going to make your feelings and situation worse. That is 100% certain, I promise you. You need professional help. Maybe a psychologist or social worker to talk to and work out your problems. If it is bad enough, perhaps a psychiatrist to put you on some medications. Your friends and even your family may scorn your decision to seek outside help beyond them. Forget the stigmatization. You have to deal with it now before it gets worse. The suicide statistics in America for youth are scary. So, do yourself a favor: if you do feel down and sad, even suicidal, for a long period of time, get some professional help. The good thing is there is nowhere else to go but 'up' at that point. You can start by talking to the school nurse or guidance counselor.

Your mind is what your whole body is centered upon. What you put into your mind will determine who you are and who you will become. Be careful and gentle with your mind.

Chapter XIII – Keeping It Real

There are two things to know for this and the next chapter that you first need to understand before you read them: 1. You were born with something 'wrong with you', and 2. Your life is not your own.

Let's start with the latter part of that sentence. (The first part will be dealt with in the next and final chapter). My father was 42 years old when he took his own life, leaving four lost kids (I was the eldest, at 12 years old) and a devastated wife. The epitaph on his gravestone reads like this:

LEO SIGMUND NEWMAN
August 22, 1935 – May 21, 1979

There is really no need for you to know his name (who names their kid 'Sigmund' anyway?), I know. And the dates are meaningless to you and anyone else. What I want you to notice about what is typed above is the smallest part in the writing: the 'dash' between my father's birthdate and the date of his death. Like him, you and everyone else who has ever, or will ever, live has a 'dash' in between these two dates. That 'dash' means something special. It is called 'Your Life'. For simplicity sakes, accept that your life that you live doesn't belong to you. No, it really doesn't. It belongs to God. My father ended his life at a young age. What he lived during that 'dash' was between him and God. In the same way, your 'dash', the way you live your life, will be between you and God. Make no mistakes about it. This simple idea is crucial towards having a happy and joy-filled life in a way that makes you special.

Quick! Do you know *the Secret to True, Lasting Happiness*?

Did you say, "a Ferrari"? Or "a million dollars"? Or "having sex with a hot girl"?

You guessed wrong, little brother! These and other *worldly* loves will help you feel good for the moment, but this good feeling will be temporary and unfulfilling. They will not lead you to the Greatest Happiness. Only one thing, and one thing alone, will make you happy and joyful all of the days of your life. That secret is… (drum-roll please!) …**Thankfulness to God**. Being Thankful to God is the highest honor you can show your Creator. It is something He deserves from you 100%. Yes, the 'Secret to Happiness' really is that easy! You must choose to be thankful to God. So, do it! Without question or hesitation!

But what can I be thankful for? You don't know how hard my life is, Mr. Michael!

Little friend, I want you to know deep inside your heart that you have so very much to be thankful to God for in life. Even right now at this very moment you can be thankful, no matter how bad your circumstances really are or appear to be. The following is just a brief list compiled from the suggestions of many good, Godly men who have counseled me over the years. The men themselves are thankful for the same things, as they know the importance of each in and throughout their lives.

Your Faith: God gives you Faith in Him. Without God, what is the point? If there is no life after death, what is the point? All scientists will tell you that you cannot destroy energy or matter or even information, but how many of us choose to believe that we also go on as Spirit after this life? Some people, even very smart and highly-educated people, in history have thought that you live in a very small piece of time and then it is all black or not even that, only nothingness, for eternity. Is that what you believe? Or do you have Faith that your life is eternal? For existence to be meaningful, give thanks for your Faith that there is a God and that all people have the option to seek eternal life. Have faith in God and you will be a happier and stronger person for your belief. Some people have hope without faith, but you cannot have faith without hope. See the world around you and believe in Him.

Your health: Okay, I am indeed making a presumption here, because you may not be in the best of health right now. You may have some physical deformity that prevents you from playing sports, or from being able to hold a pen to write with, or from being able to type on a computer keyboard. But until this book comes out in Braille or as an audio-book (and I do hope it does someday, if I can do anything about that) for the blind boys to be able to learn from it, then you have something the blind boys don't have: eyesight that allows you to read. If someone is reading this book to you, then you have the power of hearing to be thankful for. To paraphrase a line from one of my favorite songs by *The Police*: Every breath you take and every move you make, God will be watching over you. You are alive at this very moment, my friend. That is one amazing fact, isn't it? Each and every breath you take should not be taken for granted, as your life can end at any time God so chooses. I don't say this to put 'the fear of death' into you, but to put 'awe of life' into you. Life is fantastic, it's a blessing, it's wonderful, it's mysterious, and no one can create life except our Creator Himself. So, give Thanks to God that you are alive at this very moment - living and breathing, reading or listening to this book.

Your Education: You can read this book. You can speak and understand spoken English. Those are skills that you have learned which should not to be taken lightly. (Go ahead and pat yourself on the back!) These skills are highly valued in this world and set you apart from many people who have not or cannot acquire such skills. There are roughly one billion people on earth who speak English as their first or second language, with another billion and a half trying to learn English right now. Those numbers may seem big, but that really comes down to less than two people out of seven on earth can speak or write or understand English. English is the language of international relations, business, politics, and law. So, knowing English is a great advantage that you have that no one can ever take from you. Knowing how to speak proper English opens doors to many opportunities. It is also something to be thankful for in that you can read this book (which I hope is helping you a lot). Someone in your past, either a teacher or someone else, cared enough about you to teach you how to read. That is something to be really and truly thankful for. There are many people even in Western Civilization who cannot read a simple one-line sentence in whatever their native language is. They are functionally illiterate. But you have the skill to read, and maybe even the creativity inside you to write wonderful things for others to read. The same goes for other parts of your education. Like math. Can you count your change from a purchase at the convenience store? Then you are almost guaranteed a good starting job in your life because of this math skill. Albert Einstein, probably the greatest genius the world has ever known, could not count his own change when he bought something.

Patriotism: Without your country, you would be subject to attack at any time by those people, both foreign and domestic, who think they have more power than you. There are evil men all over the world who would love to destroy America. The Vikings ransacked parts of Europe repeatedly because for a long time those poor people of the land had little, or no, government to protect them. History is full of "might makes right". Hopefully you agree this is the wrong way to live, but many men (and a few women) subscribe to this belief. Your great country protects you and your rights, and you should appreciate that fact. Many men and women throughout the history of Western Civilization, and especially in the United States of America, gave up their lives willingly so you now can be free to believe what you want, act (lawfully) the way that you want, and say liberally what you want. Give thanks for those men and women who died for your freedom. Even today there are many men and women in uniform around the world and in your neighborhood sacrificing themselves for you. If you happen to meet someone who is in the military, say a strong and meaningful 'Thank You!' to them. Say 'Thank You!' to God for these people. Without them, life and freedom would not be worth much in our society, and both would most likely have disappeared long before you were born. Your country also gives you many good gifts like roads to drive on, schools to get an education from, inspectors for food safety, and police officers to stop others from drinking and driving or doing other dangerous behaviors. Your government also guarantees you many rights and freedoms that are not present in other countries, like the ability to talk trash about your country's President or your town's local Mayor. Without a doubt, we in North America live in the most just, free, and best countries in history. It is therefore only right that we should support and love our country and show respect to the people who have died to keep it, and us, safe from harm. In the same manner, show respect to flag of your country.

Other people: Almost always there is something to be gained from every relationship you build. Every person you meet in life knows something that you don't. That is like saying every person you meet is an expert on something you are not, and you can only learn from them if you give them the time and chance to teach you. One of the best and most enjoyable things in life (even if you feel yourself more to be an introvert like I am) is meeting other people for the first time and then becoming an integral part of their lives. People are awesome. People are incredible. And people all around the vast world are interested in you! Stay interested in them! Help them! All people have problems. Some people have problems with no solutions. Maybe all you can do is listen. That is still more help than many other people will do. Be thankful you have the ability to help others with their problems.

Being Thankful to God for even the littlest things will reap rewards now and, in your life, later on. Our God deserves it, and your heart will be more open and fuller of energy for it.

Chapter XIV - The Last Word Is THE WORD

"In the beginning was the Word. The Word was with God, and the Word was God." – Opening Verse in The Book of John (The Bible, NIV)

Saint Josephine Bakhita, a child slave in Africa in the late 1800s, was so young when she was abducted that she did not even know her own name. But even as a horribly tortured little girl, when she looked up to the skies, and saw the magnificence of the sun, moon, and stars, she wondered what Great Master there was Who made everything and everyone. Josephine believed in God when no one had even told her about Him. Eventually by God's Grace she was saved from slavery to become a Catholic sister. After her death, she was canonized as a Catholic Saint. A marvel she was in her life.

Here's a powerful statistic for you: The chances of anyone and everyone dying at some point in their life is 100%.

Silly for me to say, right? Okay, all silliness aside, what I am trying to say is this: Not one minute more of your life is ever guaranteed, let alone a day or more. So, would you say that making the most important decision of your life needs to be talked about here, just in the slight case your life comes to a (sadly) premature end? *What is that decision*? It's an easy decision, little brother, as you will see below, but it takes belief on your part. It's not right, but there are far too many who have lived in our time and in the world's history that have failed in this decision. As was seen at the beginning of the last chapter, you were born with something 'wrong' with you that needs to be 'fixed'. To be 100% honest with you, there is only One Way to fix that broken part of you.

The decision: TO ACCEPT JESUS CHRIST INTO YOUR HEART AS LORD AND SAVIOR.

Can you do that, my friend? Right now? Take few really deep breaths and think about it a moment if you have to. Go with your gut feelings. If you need a little guiding help, here is what is known as **The Sinner's Prayer** which will help you as you make the Right Decision. If this is your first time ever reading it, see if you can open your heart and your mind as you read it with interest. Read it out loud boldly if you can.

God My Father, I now believe that you created me out of Your Love. In many ways I have sinned against You and others. I repent of all of my sins past and present. Please forgive me. Thank You for sending your Son Jesus to die for me, to save me from hell. I choose this very day to renew a new Covenant with you and to place Jesus at the center of my heart. I surrender to Jesus as Lord over my whole life. I ask you now, God the Father, to flood my heart and soul with Your Holy Spirit and to grant me the gift of new life. Give me Your Grace and Courage to live for You alone for the rest of the days of my life. Amen.

Did you read/say that prayer? Did you say it with conviction in your mind and honest belief in your heart? Then trust that you are a Saved Person by the Grace of Christ, and that nothing can ever take away your Salvation! Eternal heaven is assured for you!

Okay, I believe in Jesus and I am saved. But what does that mean for me from now on?

Your life will be forever changed. You are a Born-Again Christian! First, you go join a Christian church and get yourself baptized (if you haven't been already) by a minister, preacher, or priest. The clergy will explain to you why baptism is important. Your faith in Jesus needs to be nurtured to grow and mature. This will not happen overnight but will take a lifetime to achieve. You need a group of Godly brothers and sisters to surround you and love you to keep you accountable for all your actions in your life. You will keep them accountable for their actions. By the way, if you are looking and waiting for the 'perfect' church to join, let me tell you that you will never find it, because all churches are imperfect. Find one where you feel you fit in and that you enjoy the ministries available to you. Over my years as a Born-Again Christian, I have attended many different Bible studies and ministry groups with leaders having different leading styles – one even in Paris, France for a short time. Some of the groups were both men and women. Some of them were just for men. Some were better (and more interesting) than others, but all of them focused on learning about only three things: Jesus Christ Our Savior, the Bible, and how our lives can be changed.

Revelation from God is progressive and lasts a lifetime. Your 'sin nature' is going to fight your desire to better yourself every step of your life's journey with God. Only Jesus can help you fight back. Don't allow yourself to be led astray by negative voices, bad urges and unholy temptations, or other pulls that will take you off-track. You must practice faith and discipline to stay on the narrow path of a Godly Life. Rely on your Christian brothers and sisters to keep you on the Narrow Road that leads to Eternal Life. Meet regularly with other Godly boys and men who have the same desire as you to walk with the Lord. Take the time daily to have personal self-study in the Bible. Pray by talking to Jesus just as you would talk to any of your homies, because Jesus will always be your most Faithful and Best Friend. All this will ultimately lead to a more fulfilling and satisfying life for you.

Change. Much of this book was about change. Hopefully all of it will be change for the better. Coming to this final point in the book, it must be noted that any permanent change in your life can only be done with the help of Jesus, God's Only Begotten Son, who died for you. Pure willpower on your own can only work for so long, maybe a few months if you are lucky. For true and long-lasting change to happen, you have to call upon the Saving Power of Jesus to make that change in you. Remember the opening quote from Jeremy Sly, the prisoner, at the beginning of this book? He accepted Christ, but it was too late for him to have freedom in this world (only) in that he was already sentenced to a lifetime in prison. But it wasn't too late for him in that he now leads many other prisoners to Belief in Jesus through performing educational duties within his prison. He has made a change in his life, and he gives thanks to the Guiding Help of Jesus. You will still encounter troubles even as a Believer for as long as you are alive. That is certain and unavoidable. However, you now have new 'tools' to deal with adversity: The Power of Jesus, Prayer to Him, and His Word (The Biblical Scriptures).

GRACE

Showing empathy, the ability to understand another's pain and feel compassion for them, is what sets us apart from the animals. God has given you this ability in order to make the world a better place. For that to happen, you have to come full circle in your beliefs about God. Jesus came down from Heaven to have empathy for you. He lived a life that had all the feelings and temptations, both positive and negative, of the world inside of Him. He felt everything there is possible to feel, and he suffered every possible suffering there is to suffer. Jesus died with a suffering pain that few in history will ever suffer. This He did all for you. You, in turn, in order to honor Jesus must go and show empathy to others. This is done through works of service. There are four S's that the world, your flesh, and the Evil One, want you to focus your life, your energy, and your efforts on: salary, sex, success, and status. All four of these S's are involved in the one prideful S: self. But Jesus wants you to focus on another S: service. That is what we all are called to do in this world: to serve God and our fellow man.

So, I ask you, my new brother in Christ: What are you going to do today to serve God and your family, your friends, your mentor, your community, your country, and the world? This does not mean you have to go out and start a new orphanage for family-less children or a hospital for the poor elderly. Serving does mean that from now on you have to set aside a portion of your time and resources for others' needs. You have to think of others first and yourself second. You are going to have to take positive action to serve others. You are going to have to "Love your neighbor as yourself". (What does it mean to love yourself? Remember, too, what you have learned in this book to take good care of yourself – mind, body, and soul - so you can be there for others and for God.)

But I am just a young teen, what can I do to serve?

I'm glad you asked! The following is a list provided by the Roman Catholic Church to direct you to proper acts of helping others and serving God:

Spiritual Works

1. Counsel those who doubt Jesus
2. Instruct those who are uneducated
3. Correct (but not judge) the one who sins
4. Comfort those who are in pain
5. Forgive those who wrong you
6. Bear offenses against you with patience
7. Pray for the living and the dead

Physical (Corporal) Works

1. Feed those who are hungry
2. Give drink to those who are thirsty
3. Clothe those who are naked

4. Shelter the homeless (you may be able to volunteer in a homeless shelter in your town)
5. Visit those who are sick
6. Visit those who are imprisoned (You are too young to visit prisoners now, but you can ask at your church if they have a Prison Ministry with the names of prisoners to whom you can send a nice note or holiday card. Prisoners are hungry for any letters from the outside.)
7. Bury the dead (Okay, sure, both of us need to leave this last one to the professionals.)

Let me add two more to this list. "Be a friend." First, stand up and defend the weak boy, the poor girl in torn and dirty clothes with messy hair, the kid with mental health problems, who are being bullied and made fun of. Second, listen to all people, both the young and the old, who are in emotional and spiritual pain. You cannot solve all of a person's problems. It's just not possible for you to do so even if you want to. But just by taking the time to sit quietly and listen attentively you may do more than help someone have a better day – you might just save their life. Suicide rates in the United States, especially for teenagers, are scary. The person you fight for, or sit with and listen to, will be helped so very much more than you can now understand at your young age. But I guarantee that in ten years you will look back and see what a wonderful, fantastic and loving person you were to stand up and fight for them or listen patiently to them. That I am sure of, little friend.

Money, sex (with your wife), fame, luxuries… All good things when in moderation. But please, for the love of yourself, don't make these materialisms and desires the center of your life. You will only end up empty and disappointed. And I don't want that for you, little brother. No, not one bit!

Dance unto the Lord. Sing for the Lord. Do whatever it is *you* love for God. For God is Love. For Love is the Body of God. Love for other people and Love for God is your only true given purpose and meaning. That's what real life is all about. With the Love of God through His Son Jesus as your One True **Father**, your life needs nothing else, absolutely nothing else, to be perfect and complete. And I wouldn't want it any other way. Wouldn't you say the same, little brother?

Tangible (Object) Skills Every Teenage Boy Should Know:

1. Change a lightbulb (Okay, I'm starting off easy here. But have you ever tried to change a fluorescent tube bulb in a long ceiling light? It's a big hassle, even with a ladder!)
2. Use simple non-power tools: hammer a nail, use a screwdriver (Philips and flathead), use a handsaw, use a wrench (adjustable, Allen, pipe, socket, etc.), use sandpaper, use a roller to paint a room/a brush to paint trim (indoors and outdoors). Do not use a power tool unless you have been properly trained on it or you could hurt yourself seriously, or at the very least damage what you are repairing/building.
3. Use a pocket ("Swiss Army") knife safely and properly
4. Use a measuring (yard) stick; use a measuring tape
5. Use a toilet plunger (messy, yes, but an important skill in any household.)
6. Use a sewing needle and thread
7. Change a bicycle tire/fix a bicycle (you can make money with this one!)
8. Fill air into a car's tires to proper PSI
9. Change a car's flat tire
10. Vacuum a car's interior at a convenience store or car wash for an adult
11. Wash a car's exterior and not leave any sudsy residue (make money with this!)
12. Change a car's oil (remember to recycle the oil – don't just dump it) and oil filter
13. Add window-washing fluid to a car

14. Add coolant to a car's cooling system (Important: read the car's instructions and product labels carefully or you can ruin the motor.)
15. Learn how to jump-start a car. Do not try it without someone who knows how to do it showing you first the correct way.
16. Learn to drive a stick-shift (standard) car (when you are old enough to drive)
17. Use a push or power-mower and weed-trimmer to cut grass (get trained on the power equipment before you use them. you can make money with this one!)
18. Rake and bag leaves, and pull and bag weeds (again, a money-maker!)
19. Plant or replant a plant or small tree or bush
20. Cook a simple breakfast, lunch, and dinner (if all you can do is burn toast or boil water, learn from your mother, or a friend's mother, or a cookbook). This will highly impress both your mother and any girl. Even pancakes or an omelet are simple enough.
21. Build a fire in your home's fireplace and use the flu correctly
22. Cook on a Barbecue grill (plenty of books available to learn this). Impress your homies.
23. Learn how to pitch a tent and go camping with your buddies, even if it's your backyard
24. Learn how to build a fire safely when you go camping, and cook on it
25. Learn how to use canoe, kayak, and row boat paddles

26. Learn how to tie several types of knots (this is handier than you think it is)
27. Run any appliance in the home: dishwasher, clothes washer and dryer, microwave oven, blender, toaster, etc. (Note: washing dishes by hand is also a skill you should know.)
28. Learn how to use Microsoft OFFICE (especially WORD and EXCEL), or the Open Source equivalent programs
29. Learn simple coding for a PC computer, tablet, or an app for other electronic devices, or for making a website (examples: HTML, JAVA, C+)
30. Learn a 1-on-1 game/sport like tennis, ping-pong, racquetball, chess, backgammon, golf, bowling. You need to have "1 on 1" kinds of fun with your mentor and your best friend.
31. Fly a kite with a young child, and make him or her happy
32. Learn how to tie a necktie and a bow tie
33. Learn how to take care of a baby (feed a baby, change a baby's diaper, bathe a baby, clothe a baby)

Intangible Skills Every Teenage Boy Should Know:

1. Your good words are followed up with your good actions
2. Discover what you love to do, and put your heart into it
3. Learn not to give up on *something* you love, no matter the difficulties
4. Learn not to give up on *someone* you love, no matter the stress
5. Be able to define a goal by writing it down and then communicating it to someone else
6. Learn that practice does not always make perfect: *perfect practice makes perfect*
7. Learn how to care for an animal
8. Have regular chores to help the family without pay
9. Learn how to dance with a girl properly and formally
10. Learn how to swim and tread water
11. Get *The Boy Scout Handbook* and learn basic wilderness survival skills
12. Learn CPR and basic first-aid. The American Red Cross or your local community college should have classes you can take. Ask for free or reduced-price classes.
13. Learn some simple self-defense techniques because you never know... (and if you have the time and money, taking up a martial art will help you both physically and mentally.)
14. Read the USDA nutritional label on the side of any box/bottle/package of food

15. Use Google or Bing to do homework research effectively and efficiently online
16. Be able to 'shop around' on eBay, Craigslist, or other websites, if only to compare prices
17. Enter contests and games to have fun and learn excellence
18. Learn to be a gracious loser and a humble winner
19. Say "yes", "no", "please", "thank you", and "you're welcome", and mean it
20. Say "I'm sorry. I apologize humbly. Please forgive me.", and mean it (a sign of maturity)
21. Say to someone in pain, "I know you are hurting. I know you are scared. But I am here for you. Can you trust me?" and mean it (This shows your love at its finest.)
22. Volunteer at your church, or at a soup kitchen, or at a homeless shelter
23. Write "thank you" notes by hand and mail them (not typed or emailed)
24. Send Christmas (or other holiday) cards to friends and family and your mentor
25. Ask yourself before you do anything important "Who or what belief is influencing me to do this action? Am I listening to my gut instinct?"
26. Learn how to maintain a conversation by being 'an active listener'
27. Learn to be patient with yourself and others. Give both yourself and others 'enough time'
28. Learn to give freely of your time, money, and effort without expecting anything in return

29. Learn to celebrate your friends' successes and rejoice with others
30. Learn to mourn with those who mourn
31. Learn to alleviate another person's suffering (just listening is often the best idea)
32. Learn to forgive others when they wrong you (a sure sign you are a mature person)
33. Learn to care from the heart for the least of God's people – they need you!
34. Learn to befriend someone who has no friend. Learn to befriend your enemies.
35. Write a poem for your mother and grandmother on Mother's Day
36. Write a poem for a special girl
37. Shower (you are no longer a kid – you will smell bad), brush your teeth at least twice a day (morning and night), and shave regularly and keep a nice haircut
38. Learn to speak a second language (Spanish is a good one for living in the USA and not too difficult to learn. Chinese will become more important and valuable to know in the coming years. Speaking any second or third language vastly improves your job skills list and will impress employers highly.)
39. Avoid tattoos and piercings (Many of you will disagree with me on this, but it is a fact that this is just a good idea to help you get the good job you want. Employers absolutely hate tattoos and piercings.)
40. Dress to impress at all times – know casual, dressy casual, business and formal

41. Know your table manners, especially with women of all ages
42. Stand up when a woman enters the room and offer her your seat
43. Don't sweat the small stuff – it will all work its way out for the better
44. Memorize "The Lord's Prayer"
45. Pray and be thankful and grateful constantly for everything good in your life
46. And finally, memorize Scripture verses that have meaning for you as you read the Bible

Additional resources that I strongly recommend you chew on for a while and devour:

Other than the online content, any books or DVDs that you may want to learn from may be at your local library. If your local library does not have one of these media you want to explore, explain to the librarian how important this content is and ask if he or she can get it for you.

The Website: WithoutAFather.com, which can help answer questions you may have or help you to find an appropriate mentor.

Ted Talks on Ted.com or Youtube.com, especially those spoken by various motivational speakers and business/political leaders. (Seeing the Ted Talk by Nick Vujicic is a *requirement* I am placing on you, little brother. I dare you to watch Nick in this video or one of his other online motivational videos and then say you're unable to accomplish your goals and desires.)

"Game Changer" – book by NFL quarterback Kirk Cousins. Highly inspirational and Godly.

"The Passion of the Christ" – a powerful movie showing Jesus' betrayal, torture, and crucifixion. While I recommend you see it, be prepared to be shocked, because you will be.

"The Purpose Driven Life" – a popular book by Pastor Rick Warren. Hint: It's not about you, it's about God, and what you can do to make the right decisions to live for Him.

"Boundaries" – a book by Stephen Arterburn (New Life Live). This book will help you learn how to set appropriate boundaries to protect yourself and maintain good relationships with others. There are many books by New Life Live that you can explore and learn from.

"Every Man's Battle" – a book by Stephen Arterburn (New Life Live) dealing with the one of the biggest sinful problems teen boys and adult men have: lust in their hearts.

"Facing the Giants" – a movie by Affirm Films. A football team and its coach have struggles and make positive and inspiring changes from within.

"War Room" – another movie by Affirm Films. All about the Power of Prayer.

"Heaven Is for Real" – A film about a young boy who goes to Heaven during an emergency operation, and lives to tell about it.

"Courageous" – possibly best seen when you are a little older. Another movie by Affirm Films about correct and appropriate fatherhood.

"Fireproof" – again, a film probably best seen when you are a little older. Another movie by Affirm Films about correct and appropriate ways a husband behaves and treats his wife in a God-centered marriage.

Any books or online videos by John Eldredge. Highly recommended for you to understand true manhood and masculinity. It is especially beneficial to read Eldredge's books as part of a group of other boys at church or with your friends for discussion.

"The Book of Man: Readings on the Path to Manhood" – by William Bennett. Title says it all.

"Chicken Soup for the Teenage Soul (series)" – Several books by Jack Canfield with inspirational stories about other teenagers and their issues for you to learn from.

"The Seven Habits of Highly Effective People" – a book by Stephen Covey. Title explains it.

The Website: TheArtofManliness.com – for understanding and learning about being a man.

"The Total Money Makeover" – a popular book by Dave Ramsey which will help you understand money and the different methods and reasons for managing it successfully.

"Your Money or Your Life" – book by Joe Dominguez. Often cited as the best book to learn money management principles from.

"How to Win Friends and Influence People" – famous book by Dale Carnegie. Title says it all.

Google the poem *Desiderata* for a light-hearted view of living a good, Godly life.

And finally, of course, **The Bible**. Life's "Big Book of Instructions". You are never wasting your time if you are reading The Bible. Or, better yet, memorizing Scripture verses from it. Do it daily and watch your life change. GetAFreeBible.com will send you a paperback copy for free if you can't afford to buy one.

Resources Online and On the Phone to Help You

1-800-RUNAWAY the National Runaway Hotline. Also, www.1800Runaway.org. A phone number and website in case you find yourself being a teen runaway (though I advise against it) and you need immediate help. 24 hours a day / 365 days a year.

1-800-656-HOPE National sexual assault hotline. If you are ever sexually assaulted.

www.acf.hhs.gov/programs/fysb/content/youthdivision/pro grams/sopfactsheet.htm A website for street outreach for you to get in contact with if you need assistance.

www.lsc.gov/find-legal-aid If you are in trouble with the law and need legal assistance.

www.servicelocator.org/libraries.asp A website to help you find your closest local library for materials listed in this book or for other reading and listening media you may be interested in.

1-800-780-2294 A phone number for you to connect with a substance or alcohol abuse counselor if you have an addiction or problem. You can also check out their website www.samhsa.gov

apps.unitedway.org/myuw   Website for the United Way charitable organization which can help you find resources or help you in many ways to meet your needs. You can also call 211 on the phone to reach someone who may be able to help you.

1-800-273-TALK The suicide-prevention hotline. Call them 24 hours a day / 365 days a year if you ever feel suicidal and have nowhere else to turn.

www.icphusa.org Institute for Children, Poverty, and Homelessness. A good resource for assistance if you or your family become homeless.

A Final Note Before We Come to Closure

So? So! Here we are, little man. The end of the book. Where are we now? Have you learned anything that you think can help you on your journey to becoming a *Real Man* in this world we have been put in by a loving God? That is my one true hope for you now and always. And I also hope you will keep coming back to this book for further guidance and information, such as to look up a website or advice that can help you again later on. That brings us to the end, yes, but before I close out, let me add just a few small thoughts which I definitely think need to be said (or repeated again).

Writing down your life story. Some people call this *journaling* or *keeping a diary*. Put your life experiences, the negatives ones especially, down on paper (or type them into a computer document) that you can come back to later and read again. This will help you to see where you have been, how it all got you to where you are now, and what you can change to make life better for you in the future. Writing a page a day is excellent, but you need not be so diligent. Try to write at least a page a week. Believe me, it will do wonders for your outlook on life as you learn from your own experiences, mistakes and all.

Social Media. If you do Facebook, Kik, Instagram, Snapchat, or any other social media applications or websites on the internet, know full well, my friend that your desired college is going to research you online. Anything negative, such as a picture of you drinking beer half-naked with your homies, is going to show up and work against you. The same goes for future employers.

Increasingly employers are going online to research job applicants, and you can be sure they will find out anything and everything they can about you online. The internet is useful for storing information, but it is also a permanent catalogue of anything you place on it, and that has the possibility to make it very dangerous. If you put any picture or statement, no matter how innocent, out there on the internet, know that you can never get that back. You cannot fully erase what you post. It will always be on the internet, and it will haunt you for the rest of your life. So please, be careful and be wise when using social media, blogs, comment sections, and other parts of the internet to place your information. It will cost you down the road if you are placing obscene or negative material on the internet. You can be sure of that 100%. In the same regard, be respectful of other people, especially girls who can be preyed upon by bad men, when posting content or pictures.

If you want a friend, be a friend. There is no other way for friendship to happen. Only babies get unconditional love. You are going to have to put the time and effort and love into a friendship to get something in return. Don't waste your life pursuing things that don't matter. Don't even think about things that don't matter as that is a waste of time in itself. Research shows that a long, happy life that a 'lucky' person has is always marked by having good, solid relationships built on love, trust, and mutual respect. This goes for all your relationships, from your mother, to your mentor, to your homies, to your someday wife (if you have one). If you can, find someone today who desperately *needs* a friend (like the boy being bullied in the school hallway or on the school bus), and I guarantee you will *make* and *have* a new friend for life.

Keep short accounts with people. People are going to make you angry in life. They are going to let you down many times. If you suffer from what my mother called "Irish Alzheimer's" ("forgetting everything except the grudges"), you are going to end up very alone and very lonely very quickly. Learn to forgive and move on. People in turn may or may not forgive you, but you must do your best to live at peace with all people. This is not just for your own personal emotional well-being. It is also what God commands you to do.

Learn the Art of Business. Unless you are a hermit on a desert island, business will be a part of your life all your life. Learn how to earn a dollar efficiently and easily (but legally!). Learn how to save a dime whenever you spend a dollar. Learn how to negotiate deals. You might be an aggressive negotiator, but that only works for one-off sales; you need to cultivate relationships and trust for repeat business. One idea to master for negotiating is the understanding that patience and silence can work to your advantage. Patience also gels situations in all types of personal relationships. If a lunatic is raging in your face, remaining calm and not reacting may let them yell a while, but eventually the person will realize he cannot 'own' you and will only look like a fool to people around you. Another trick for business? Humor… works very well! Get funny and make friends and customers!

Don't ever let anyone look down on you and discourage you because you are young. You have much to offer this world even at the young age you are now. Don't ever forget that! And don't limit your challenges. Instead challenge your limits. Being young is a limit, but you can rise above that. Do it and gain big time.

Be true to yourself and be yourself always and everywhere. If you want to get angry, get angry (just don't hurt anyone or break anything). If you want to pick some flowers from your garden to give to the pretty (or not so pretty) girl next door, do it, even if the other boys will laugh at you. If you say you want to study to be a preacher someday, and other boys laugh at you, ignore them, and start today by reading the Bible as much as you can. Ask anyone any question you want. The world is here for you in so many ways, little friend. Take life, take it all, as much as you want, with both hands tightly, while you can. Don't waste time because you will never be the age you are at again.

Be not afraid. Yes, the Road you are on in life is going to be a stormy one, perhaps even full of danger and turmoil. It already is a hard one for you right now as a fatherless teenage boy. *But will it always be a 'hard road'?* Yes. For sure. That will always be the case as long as you live. Trust that God the Father through His Son Jesus by the Power of the Holy Spirit will walk each and every step with you, day by day, moment by moment. He will carry you through the really difficult times when life gets hard. He will go a long way to making that hard road easier for you to trudge along, step by slow careful step. Be strong and bold and courageous in your faith in God. Live unafraid like no one else does because you know in your heart you can do it.

Choices. I hope that you picked up on the major theme of this book: making the right decisions. Each and every day you make thousands of choices. They all will affect you, either positively or negatively, depending on how you choose. As said above, be true to yourself and make the right choices that will benefit you now, during your entire life, and through eternity.

God's Grace is also God's Law. What happens if I'm on drugs and I believe I can fly as I step off a balcony on a high-rise building? That's right: splat dead on the sidewalk below! It's the same with God's Law. It doesn't matter what you believe: You cannot break God's Law without bad consequences. In the same way, the world will not stop for you or even stop attacking you. That's like asking a snake not to bite you or a bear not to rip you apart.

Finally, **Be here now**. The past is in the past. There is not much you can do about it now, right? The future is not yet here, so why worry about it? Be always focused on the present, wherever you are, and you will always be 'the best you' that you can be!

All the best to you, little man. Smile! Jesus loves you! From me, once a fatherless boy myself, to you-

God bless and Godspeed!

~Michael W. Newman

As with all the books I have written, sales of this book will support a chosen charity. I am choosing **Covenant House**, which is a refuge for runaway teenagers, serving in twenty-eight big cities in the United States and in six other countries. Covenant House takes teenage kids off the streets who have run away from home and can't find their way in life. If you ever find yourself in trouble at home, or if you are a runaway, Covenant House has a special phone number you can call: 1-800-999-9999. Someone on the other end of that phone line is there to help you and care for you.

63235224R00076

Made in the USA
Middletown, DE
25 August 2019